Clinical Dermatopathology

Clinical Dermatopathology
A TEXT AND COLOUR ATLAS

Alan Stevens

MB BS (Lond) FRCPath

Senior Lecturer in Pathology, University of Nottingham
Honorary Consultant Pathologist, Trent Regional Health Authority (T)

Paul R. Wheater

BA Hons (York) BMed Sci Hons (Nott) BM BS (Nott)

General Practitioner, Cambridge

James S. Lowe

BMed Sci Hons (Nott) BM BS (Nott) MRCPath

Senior Lecturer in Pathology, University of Nottingham
Honorary Consultant Pathologist, Trent Regional Health Authority (T)

CHURCHILL LIVINGSTONE
EDINBURGH LONDON MELBOURNE AND NEW YORK 1989

CHURCHILL LIVINGSTONE
Medical Division of Longman Group UK Limited

Distributed in the United States of America by Churchill
Livingstone Inc., 1560 Broadway, New York, N.Y. 10036,
and by associated companies, branches and representatives
throughout the world.

First published 1989

ISBN 0-443-02583-5

British Library Cataloguing in Publication Data

Stevens, Alan
   Clinical dermatopathology.
   1. Man. Skin. Diagnosis
   I. Title II. Wheater, Paul R. III. Lowe, James
   616.5'075

Library of Congress Cataloging in Publication Data

Stevens, Alan, MRCPath.
   Clinical dermatopathology: a text and colour atlas/Alan
Stevens, Paul Wheater, James Lowe.
   p. cm.
   1. Skin – Histopathology – Atlases.
   2. Skin – Diseases – Diagnosis – Atlases.
   I. Wheater, Paul R. II. Lowe, J.S. (James Steven)
   III. Title.
   [DNLM: 1. Skin Diseases – pathology – atlases.
   S844b]
   RL81.S67 1989
   616.5 '071' 0222-dc19

Produced by Longman Group (FE) Ltd
Printed in Hong Kong

Preface

Dermatologists are performing skin biopsies in increasing numbers in quest of an accurate tissue diagnosis as the basis for effective management of skin disease. Unfortunately they do not always get the diagnostic pathology service which they deserve.

Diagnostic dermatopathology is difficult for a number of reasons. Firstly, few skin conditions have pathognomonic histological appearances; many of those which do are easily recognised clinically, rendering biopsy unnecessary. Secondly, the spectrum of skin disorders is vast, in contrast to other epithelial surfaces, such as the gastrointestinal and urinary tracts where there is a very limited range. Thirdly, by the time most skin lesions are biopsied, they may have been subjected to a number of external agents such as trauma from scratching, and topical therapeutic agents which can modify the histological changes. Finally, and in our view the most important of all, there is an unacceptable degree of ignorance of clinical dermatology among histopathologists who are attempting to acquire diagnostic competence in dermatopathology; it is no coincidence that the best diagnostic dermatopathologists in the past (and probably currently) were experienced clinical dermatologists.

For many histopathologists inexperienced in dermatopathology, and faced with a skin biopsy, the first diagnostic manoeuvre is to attempt to find a photomicrograph with which it fits in one of the excellent and well-illustrated dermatopathology texts such as those cited below. This technique, known disparagingly as 'wallpaper matching', is the furthest that many histopathologists proceed along the path to dermatopathological competence. If no match can be found, a noncommittal and uninformative histological report follows, to the detriment of patient, dermatologist and the histopathologist's reputation. The need to rely on this empirical approach results from a combination of lack of knowledge of clinical dermatology and a failure to comprehend the basic principles of tissue changes in the skin.

In a similar, but less critical way, dermatologists who aim to acquire dermatopathological competence are sometimes hampered by a lack of basic histopathological knowledge.

Our objective in writing this book has been to provide an illustrated guide to diagnostic dermatopathology, linking the histopathological changes to the clinical appearances of lesions where informative, and where relevant (as in the chapters on vasculitis, granulomatous disease and epidermal dysplasia) to enunciate the basic histopathological principles which underlie the skin changes. The book is therefore aimed at trainee and consultant histopathologists who are inexperienced in dermatopathology and wish to gain a basic understanding of a diagnostic approach to skin problems, in the context of the clinical dermatology long forgotten from their student days. It is also intended that the book will provide dermatologists of all grades with an introduction to dermatopathology, whether their intention is to understand the pathological basis of their specialty or to become capable of carrying out their own diagnostic histology. In addition, we also hope that the clinical component, both text and photographs, will be of value to general practitioners, junior hospital staff and clinical medical students alike, as an aide memoire or even as an illustrated introduction to day-to-day dermatology. Many of the clinical photographs in this book are of patients presenting in the general practice of one of the authors (PRW), and photographed, and biopsied when relevant, by him at the time of presentation.

Nevertheless, the book is essentially concerned with the histopathology of the commonly occurring and important skin diseases; as such it is neither comprehensive nor concerned with management. For more detailed treatments of the pathology, and for discussion and illustration of less common conditions, the reader is referred to the excellent larger textbooks of dermatopathology by Lever and Ackerman, and the equally excellent but smaller books *Milne's Dermatopathology*, edited by Mackie, and *A Guide to Dermatohistopathology* by Pinkus and Mehregan. Standard dermatopathology textbooks such as these, and books dealing with current dermatological concepts and practice, for example *Textbook of Dermatology* edited by Rook et al., are excellent sources of references for all of the topics in this book.

Acknowledgements

Our greatest debt of gratitude goes to Dr Jerry Marsden, now Consultant Dermatologist at Birmingham General Hospital, for his help with some of the clinical aspects of the book and for the provision of a number of the clinical photographs. His continued interest in the project at all stages, his suggestions and criticism, are deeply appreciated. Any errors of fact, emphasis or presentation are the responsibility of the authors, for we probably ignored his advice. Dr Roger Allen of the Dermatology Department, University Hospital, Nottingham, played an important part in the conception of the book, and continued to advise us at various stages. Dr Marjorie Walker saw the early manuscript and gave us much valuable expert advice and criticism, for which we are immensely grateful. Dr Ken MacLennan read the early drafts of the chapter on lymphoma in the skin and made many helpful comments.

Paraffin sections were prepared in the Department of Pathology, University Hospital, Nottingham, by Janet Palmer, Ian Wilson and Anne Wilson, with great skill and patience. The microscope slides photographed here represent only a small fraction of the vast number of paraffin blocks which they sectioned, often at many levels, to provide a section suitable in content for photomicrography. Electron micrographs were prepared by Mr Trevor Gray, acrylic resin sections by Mr Neil Hand, and immunocytochemical slides by Mr Ken Morrell, all of the Department of Pathology, University of Nottingham; immunofluorescence illustrations were kindly supplied by Dr Richard Powell and Mr Dennis Marriott of the Department of Immunology, University of Nottingham. Mr Bill Brackenbury and Mr M.Creasey are responsible for a number of the clinical photographs.

Many fellow pathologists in Nottingham assisted by diverting to us slides of good examples of skin conditions; we are particularly grateful to Dr Peter James who generously gave us free access to his collection of skin slides, and provided us with a number of key histology slides when all seemed lost.

We wish to express our thanks to Dr Roger Allen, Dr Les Millard, Dr Eric Saihan and Dr Philip Kilby of the Dermatology Department, University Hospital, Nottingham, who kindly loaned us clinical photographs from their own collections for reproduction in this book. We are grateful to the United Medical and Dental Schools of Guy's and St. Thomas's Hospitals for permission to reproduce four clinical photographs.

Typing and word-processing were carried out with great diligence, patience and good humour by Isabella Streeter and Sharon Sharpe. The colour photomicrography was performed by one of the authors (PRW) using a Leitz Vario-Orthomat microscope.

Finally we would like to express our gratitude to our wives Chris, Valerie and Pamela for their support and their tolerance of our frequent absences from the hearth, our variations in mood, and general air of distraction during the preparation of this book.

Contents

1. Tissue diagnosis in dermatology

Histological examination of skin is of major importance in clinical dermatology, but it cannot always provide an accurate diagnosis. The histological findings should always be considered in conjunction with the clinical history, the naked-eye appearances of the lesion, and results of other investigations. There are six main reasons why a tissue diagnosis is not infallible:

1. **Non-specific histological features**: with the exception of some tumours, few dermatological conditions display pathognomonic histological features since the skin has a limited number of ways in which it can respond to damage. Thus, lesions which are quite distinct clinically may have similar histological appearances, and for this reason full clinical data is vital if the pathologist is to help. For example, if a skin biopsy which shows subepidermal bullae with a neutrophilic infiltrate (containing some eosinophils) in the bulla and the underlying upper dermis, is accompanied by a request form such as shown in Fig 1.1a the diagnosis proferred by the pathologist may include pemphigoid, dermatitis herpetiformis and erythema multiforme, to the confusion of all. If the specimen is accompanied by a request form as shown in Figure 1.1b then the accurate diagnosis of herpes gestationis can be made. Note that this latter, exemplary, request form mentions that the biopsy is of a vesicular lesion; this will ensure that the pathologist will examine *all* the biopsy material until a typical lesion is found. If no vesicle is present in the first stained section supplied by the laboratory, the tissue block can be sectioned at many levels until the vesicle appears. As well as basic items like the patient's age and sex, the nature, distribution and duration of the lesions should be mentioned, and other possibly associated clinical conditions, e.g. arthropathy, myositis, malignancy. Failure to give adequate clinical data may lead to an inaccurate or unhelpful histological report.

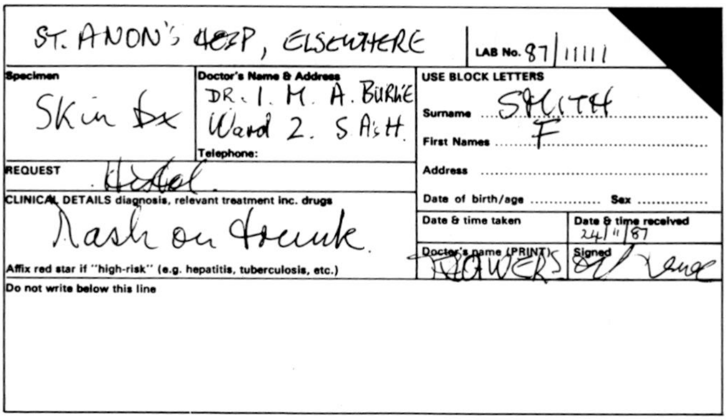
ST. ANON'S HOSP, ELSEWHERE
LAB No. 87/11111
Specimen: Skin Bx
Doctor's Name & Address: DR. I. M. A. BURKE, Ward 2. S A's H.
Telephone:
USE BLOCK LETTERS
Surname: SMITH
First Names: F
Address:
REQUEST: Histol
CLINICAL DETAILS diagnosis, relevant treatment inc. drugs: Rash on trunk.
Date of birth/age .... Sex ....
Date & time taken
Date & time received 24/11/87
Affix red star if "high-risk" (e.g. hepatitis, tuberculosis, etc.)
Doctor's name (PRINT) FLOWERS
Signed
Do not write below this line

Fig. 1.1a

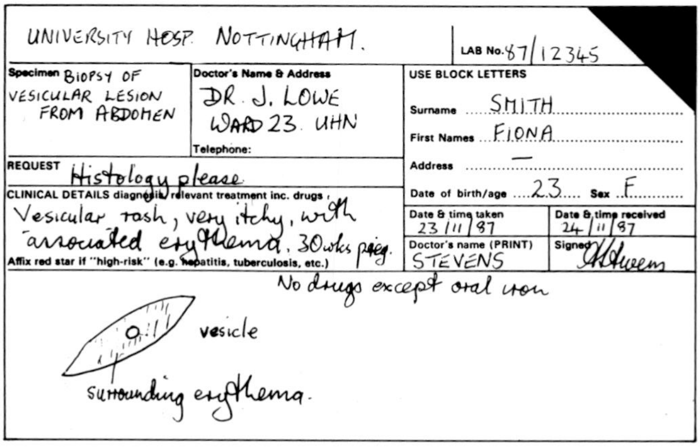
UNIVERSITY HOSP. NOTTINGHAM.
LAB No. 87/12345
Specimen: BIOPSY OF VESICULAR LESION FROM ABDOMEN
Doctor's Name & Address: DR. J. LOWE, WARD 23. UHN
Telephone:
USE BLOCK LETTERS
Surname: SMITH
First Names: FIONA
Address: —
REQUEST: Histology please
CLINICAL DETAILS diagnosis, relevant treatment inc. drugs: Vesicular rash, very itchy, with associated erythema. 30wks preg.
Date of birth/age 23 Sex F
Date & time taken 23/11/87
Date & time received 24/11/87
Affix red star if "high-risk" (e.g. hepatitis, tuberculosis, etc.)
Doctor's name (PRINT) STEVENS
Signed
No drugs except oral iron

Fig. 1.1b

2. **Atypical lesions**: dermatologists rarely require histological examination of easily diagnosed, classical skin lesions; the usual indication for biopsy is uncertainty about the diagnosis, often because of atypical features in the clinical appearances or in the history and progress of the lesion. Lesions which are clinically atypical will almost certainly be histologically atypical, since the clinical appearance is dependent on the pathological changes occurring in the lesion. In these circumstances it is important for the pathologist to have not only the clinical data, but also the dermatologist's differential diagnoses. Even if the pathologist cannot make a definite histological diagnosis, he may well be able to exclude one or more of the suggested differential diagnoses.

3. **Natural history of skin lesions**: the histological appearances of most skin lesions vary according to their stage of development. Most of the classical descriptions of dermatohistopathology are of florid lesions, biopsied at the height of their activity; lesions biopsied at an early stage of their development may show entirely different non-specific changes, as may lesions close to resolution or modified by treatment or trauma. Therefore biopsy of florid active lesions usually provides the greatest chance of accurate histological diagnosis. An exception is in the blistering diseases where the florid lesion may be too advanced (or modified by secondary changes) to be of value diagnostically; in such cases a biopsy of a very early lesion is usually required.

4. **Selection of lesion to be biopsied**: the lesion selected for biopsy should be typical of the condition as a whole. This is largely a matter of experience, enhanced by an adequate knowledge of the histopathology of the condition under investigation. Lesions which are likely to be modified histologically by, for example, trauma or unsuccessful topical treatment, should not be biopsied.

5. **Use of the appropriate biopsy technique**: the biopsy may be uninterpretable because an inappropriate biopsy technique has been used. Details of the various methods of obtaining biopsy samples of skin are given in the next chapter, but a few principles can be outlined here. First of all, pathologists abhor curette biopsies which often only succeed in scraping off the overlying keratin from lesions such as seborrhoeic keratoses. Any scanty fragments of epidermis obtained are extensively 'diluted' by keratin and the biopsy fragments are impossible to orientate in the laboratory (see Ch. 2) for the production of suitable interpretable histological sections; the laboratory may have to sample the tissue block at many levels to ensure the presence of epidermis in the diagnostic slides. This is time-consuming and frequently fruitless. There may be therapeutic indications for removing a lesion by curette, never diagnostic ones. Similarly, biopsies containing only epidermis and upper dermis are useless if the lesion is deep dermal or subcutaneous. It is also important for the dermatologist to remember that a lesion which is blatantly obvious when in situ, by virtue of erythema, swelling, petechiae etc., becomes virtually invisible when the biopsy has been fixed in formalin, since nearly all colour disappears into a characterless creamy-grey uniformity. The tissue shrinks and hardens with the result that small papules may become undetectable to the naked eye, and localized areas of induration become indistinguishable. The danger is that the inexperienced pathologist will not submit the correct part of the biopsy sample for processing, the lesion being cut away during trimming of the tissue prior to processing. Methods of avoiding this are discussed in Chapter 2, but a simple sketch on the request form, such as given in Figure 1.1b, can be of great help.

6. **Correct handling of biopsy sample**: many specialized histological techniques can now be applied to tissue biopsies, and increasing numbers of laboratories are able to offer these facilities. The more common of these techniques, and their possible diagnostic value in dermatopathology, are briefly outlined in Chapter 2. The clinician's concern is to ensure that the specimen reaches the laboratory in a state suitable for the relevant technique to be applied. In summary, routine paraffin and thin acrylic resin sections require fixation in formalin. Immunofluorescence, enzyme histochemistry and some immunohistochemical methods require fresh, unfixed tissue from which frozen sections can be prepared. Frozen sections should *never* be requested on suspected mycobacterial lesions; one biopsy sample should be submitted to the histopathology laboratory in abundant formalin fixative, and a separate piece sent fresh and unfixed to the microbiology laboratory for culture. Tissues submitted for electron microscopy should preferably be placed in an appropriate fixative, usually buffered glutaraldehyde, although ultrastructural preservation may be satisfactory when buffered formalin has been used for transportation to the laboratory, providing the biopsy sample is transferred to a more suitable fixative immediately on arrival. Hairs for scanning electron microscopy can be sent dry.

2. The skin biopsy–methods and laboratory handling

The following methods are available for obtaining a sample of skin for histological examination:
1. Excisional or incisional biopsy using a scalpel;
2. Punch biopsy;
3. Curette biopsy;
4. Shave biopsy.

Excisional or incisional scalpel biopsy

An ellipse of skin is excised under local anaesthesia and removed using a skin hook to avoid forceps damage.

Figure 2.1 shows a typical *excision biopsy*, with the lesion at the centre of the ellipse. This method is suitable for most small skin tumours, for medium-sized macules, papules and for blisters of most types. Since the lesion may become less obvious after fixation, it is important that the lesion be located at the centre of the ellipse to facilitate accurate trimming and sectioning of the biopsy in the laboratory. For the removal of a tumour, the biopsy should be deep and wide enough to ensure complete excision. When the lesion is in deep dermis or subcutis, these regions should be included in the biopsy, although it is preferable to include subcutis in all biopsies.

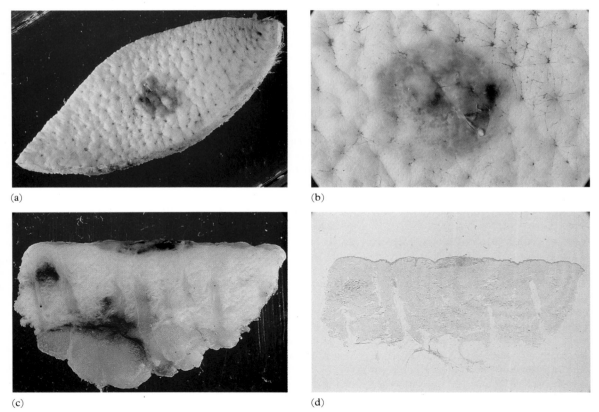

(a)   (b)

(c)   (d)

Fig. 2.1 (a)–(d) Excisional biopsy
(a) shows a typical excision biopsy specimen of a suspicious melanocytic lesion. Note the width of excision. (b) shows the same lesion after formalin fixation and colour restoration in alcohol, photographed under the dissecting microscope. Note the variation in pigmentation and ill-defined boundaries. (c) shows the lesion transected after fixation to provide a flat, vertical representative face for sectioning. (d) shows the histological section prepared from the specimen.

A typical *incision biopsy* is shown in Figure 2.2, approximately one half of the sample being lesional skin, the other normal skin. This technique is used when the lesion is too large for excision biopsy, or prior to complete surgical excision of, for example, a tumour. It may also be used for the diagnosis of blistering disorders, when the perilesional skin is sent for direct immunofluorescent examination.

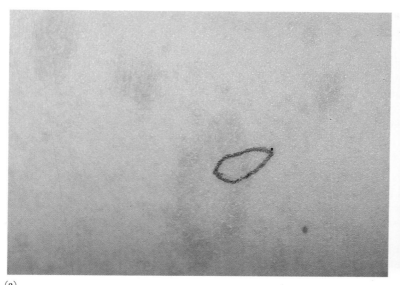
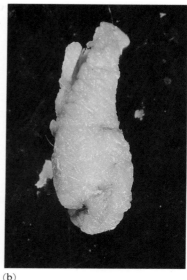

(a)   (b)

Fig. 2.2 (a) & (b) Incisional biopsy
(a) shows the clinical lesion in situ, a suspected oval 'herald' patch of pityriasis rosea. The proposed incision biopsy site is marked; note that the biopsy is to include normal surrounding skin, the peripheral scaling collarette and some of the central pink macular area. (b) shows the biopsy sample after 12 hours in formalin fixative; note that the loss of colour during fixation has led to loss of distinction between normal and erythematous skin. The shrinkage and distortion produced by fixation causes the specimen to curl and can make embedding difficult unless the biopsy is trimmed as shown in Figure 2.8(b). Failure to trim such a specimen leads to production of oblique sections.

Punch biopsy

The use of a disposable 3–4 mm diameter punch is a convenient way of obtaining a sample of skin for histological examination. If the lesion is small and focal it is important that it is at the centre of the punch, but punch biopsies can also be used to sample large lesions.

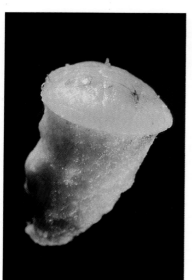

Fig. 2.3. Punch biopsy
This figure shows a typical punch biopsy specimen after fixation; note that it contains epidermis, dermis and a little subcutis. The epidermal roughening can be seen in this fixed specimen in which the colour has been restored with alcohol, using a dissecting microscope or powerful magnifier.

The commonest faults with punch biopsies are the use of too small a punch and inadequate depth of penetration. Punch biopsies are usually too small to permit samples to be trimmed off in the unfixed state for possible electron microscopy, but trimming is possible when the biopsy specimen has hardened after fixation; it is even easier when the specimen has been fixed and partly dehydrated in alcohol. The punch biopsy must be handled with extreme gentleness during its removal, taking care to produce no crush artefact by using forceps. This is easiest if the biopsy penetrates the entire dermis through to subcutaneous fat.

Curetted tissue

Superficial lesions such as seborrhoeic warts can be removed by curette, although the material obtained is usually unsatisfactory for adequate histological examination. All the material must be embedded in paraffin wax and often needs to be sectioned at many levels to ensure that epidermis is included; curetted tissue is impossible to orientate properly for histological sectioning, and so is often uninterpretable. There is the risk that an over-helpful pathologist may proffer an inaccurate diagnosis on this unsatisfactory material; curette biopsies are discouraged.

Shave biopsies

This technique is frequently used to remove benign intradermal melanocytic naevi, but can be used to provide tissue for histological diagnosis prior to definitive excision of some neoplasms.

In many cases, shave biopsies produce an adequate skin sample for histological diagnosis, but should only be used when the lesion is obviously superficial, since these biopsies usually comprise only epidermis and upper dermis.

Laboratory handling of skin biopsies

The following techniques are available for the histological examination of skin biopsies:

1. **Paraffin sections** cut at 3–5 µm thickness and stained with haematoxylin and eosin (H & E) are adequate for histological diagnosis in most cases; a wide range of special stains can be applied, the most useful of which are given in Table 2.1. The biopsy should be fixed in a formalin fixative.

2. **Acrylic (usually glycol methacrylate) resin sections** cut at 1–2 µm give greater cellular detail and better resolution. They are particularly useful when high magnification is required, e.g. for the identification of viral inclusions (see Fig. 2.4(b)). The biopsy may be fixed in formalin or, if small, in the glutaraldehyde or paraformaldehyde fixative used for electron microscopy. Haematoxylin and eosin is the most frequently used stain, but most of the special stains used with paraffin sections can be applied to glycol methacrylate sections with some modifications.

3. **Histochemistry** almost always requires frozen sections cut at 5–8 µm on a cryostat. The diagnostic value of enzyme histochemistry in dermatopathology has not been fully explored, although the chloroacetate esterase method is an excellent mast cell stain for use on frozen sections, and the same enzyme (demonstrated using the pararosanilin method) can be applied to paraffin sections to demonstrate neutrophils and neutrophil precursors (e.g. in myeloid leukaemic infiltrates) as well as mast cells. Lipid histochemical methods may be used to demonstrate lipid material in histiocytoma (see Fig. 2.5(b) and the abnormal stored glycolipid in vascular endothelium in Fabry's disease.

4. **Immunofluorescence methods** may be of considerable diagnostic value in some skin disorders. Two basic methods exist: direct and indirect techniques. In *direct* immunofluorescent methods, specific fluorescein-labelled antisera (usually against immunoglobulins, complement components or fibrin) are applied to fresh frozen sections of a patient's skin, and viewed under a fluorescence microscope, preferably one which uses epi-illumination. Localization within the skin is demonstrated by bright green fluorescence; the nature and distribution of the immunoreactants present may suggest a specific diagnosis (see Figs. 2.6(a), 8.10, 8.12). In *indirect* immunofluorescent methods, a patient's serum is applied to a fresh frozen section of a non-specific squamous epithelium such as monkey oesophagus; any circulating antibody in the serum binds to the specific sites on the substrate tissue, and are then visualized by the application of fluorescein-labeled antisera. Indirect immunofluorescent techniques thus demonstrate circulating antibodies which have the potential for localization in skin, whereas direct immunofluorescence demonstrates the antibodies in situ. In general, direct methods are more valuable as a specific aid to diagnosis. Immunofluorescent methods are valuable in blistering diseases (see Ch. 8) and in some connective tissue disorders (see Ch. 9).

5. **Immunohistochemical methods** are in their infancy in dermatopathological diagnosis but they have immense potential. An example of their use is shown in Figure 2.6(b). Although some techniques using specific monoclonal antibodies require unfixed frozen sections, many useful immunohistochemical methods can be applied to formalin-fixed paraffin sections. Immunohistochemical methods are particularly valuable in the investigation of lymphocytic infiltrations of the skin and cutaneous T cell lymphoma (see Ch. 22).

6. **Electron microscopy** is of particular value in the diagnosis of viral lesions (Fig. 10.1(f)), tumours such as Cutaneous T cell lymphoma (see Fig. 22.1) and Merkel cell tumours, Fabry's disease (Fig. 21.3(b)), and in the classification of the various types of epidermolysis bullosa (Fig. 8.9(b)). Biopsy samples should be small, contain a minimum of non-lesional skin, and be fixed in buffered glutaraldehyde or paraformaldehyde. In some cases it is possible to obtain satisfactory electron microscopy using fragments dug out of a paraffin block and reprocessed into an epoxy resin.

Scanning electron microscopy may be useful in the examination of abnormal hair types, but has otherwise found little general diagnostic application in dermatopathology.

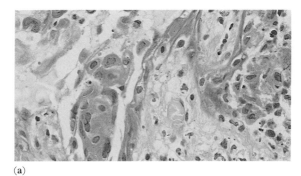

(a)

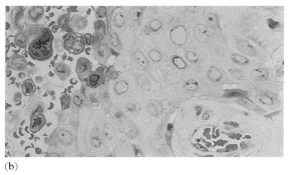

(b)

Fig. 2.4(a) & (b). Paraffin and Glycol methacrylate sections: a comparison
Figure 2.4(a) shows a routine paraffin 5 μm section stained with H & E to show viral inclusions in keratinocyte nuclei in shingles; (b) shows the same lesion in an H & E-stained

2 μm section prepared from tissue embedded in glycol methacrylate resin. Note the greater clarity of the resin section, in particular the excellent structural detail of normal and degenerate keratinocytes and of the intranuclear viral inclusions.

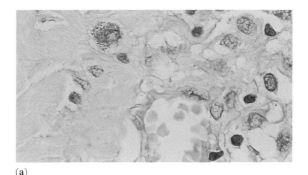

(a)

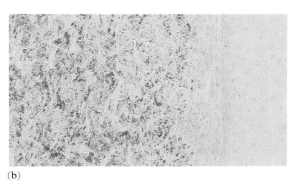

(b)

Fig. 2.5(a) & (b) Enzyme and lipid histochemical methods
Fig. 2.5(a) demonstrates the use of chloroacetate esterase in the identification of mast cells in skin. The mast cell

granules are bright red; (b) demonstrates the use of the Oil Red O technique to show fine lipid droplets in a histiocytoma in the skin.

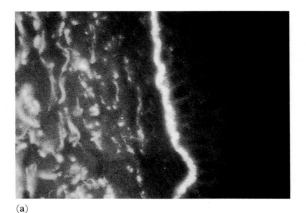

(a)

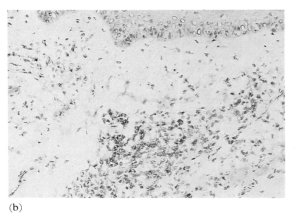

(b)

Fig. 2.6(a) & (b). Immunofluorescent and immunocytochemical methods

Fig. 2.6(a) demonstrates the use of an immunofluorescent method. Here linear basement membrane staining for IgG is seen in the skin of a patient with SLE (see Ch. 9).

(b) demonstrates the use of immunoperoxidase methods. Here, T cells are identified as the predominant component of a heavy lymphocytic infiltrate of the skin, suggesting a diagnosis of cutaneous T cell lymphoma.

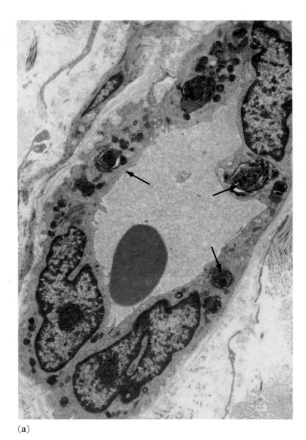

(a)

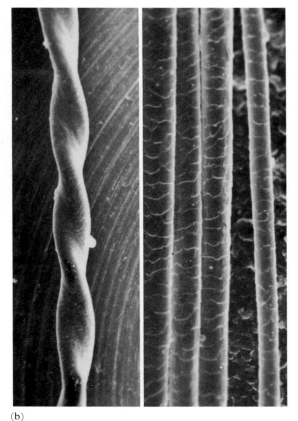

(b)

Fig 2.7(a) & (b). Ultrastructural Methods

In Figure 2.7(a) the presence of electron-dense inclusions (arrows) in the endothelial cells in dilated upper dermal capillaries confirms the diagnosis of angiokeratoma corporis diffusum (Fabry's disease).

Figure 2. 7(b) demonstrates one of the rare diagnostic applications of scanning electron microscopy in skin disease. The twisted hair (pili torti) is typical of the hereditary disorder, Menke's syndrome; normal hair is included for comparison.

Blocking of skin biopsies

Careful blocking and sectioning of a skin biopsy is a vital prerequisite to accurate histological diagnosis; imprecise orientation at paraffin embedding may make a good biopsy histologically uninterpretable. The aim should be to produce a histological section which represents a vertical slice down through epidermis, dermis and subcutis, at right angles to the epidermal surface. Obliquity may lead to a greatly distorted appearance, particularly of the epidermis, dermo-epidermal junction and dermal papillae.

Excision and Incision biopsies

Obliquity is particularly a problem in small excision or incision scalpel biopsies, since there is a natural tendency for the biopsy to be broad at the epidermal surface but narrow down at the lower margin, and to have sloping sides. If such a specimen is embedded without trimming it will be lain flat along one long sloping side, and this will be the angle at which it is sectioned; with each deeper section, the plane of sectioning remains irretrievably oblique; see Figure 2.8(a). This leads to a number of problems; in particular the architecture at the dermo-epidermal junction can be grossly distorted, giving a false impression of epidermal thickening, and leading to confusion when it is important to assess whether there is early invasion of a tumour across the epidermal basement membrane (e.g. as in superficial spreading malignant melanoma; see Fig. 19.10). It is also impossible to produce an accurate measurement of the depth of invasion of a tumour, for example the Breslow thickness of malignant melanoma. This obliquity can be avoided by trimming off (with a sharp razor blade under dissecting microscope control) one edge of the biopsy to provide a flat vertical face for sectioning; all subsequent deeper levels will be properly orientated; see Figure 2.8(b). The trimmed fragment may be saved for subsequent electron microscopy or embedding in acrylic resin. When the biopsy is large and contains an easily visible central lesion, the above trimming should remove about one-third of the lesion, leaving two-thirds to be included in the processed block. This allows a representative histological section of the main body of the lesion to be achieved with minimal trimming on the microtome, and allows a small piece of reserve tissue to be stored for other purposes.

In many excision biopsies for tumour, e.g. basal cell carcinoma, it is vital to determine histologically whether the lesion has been completely excised, and in such cases, accurate block selection and trimming is even more important; wrong block selection can give a false impression that the lesion has been completely excised. When lateral clearance of excision of a tumour must be confirmed, it is useful to take 'cruciate' blocks (see Fig. 2.9(a)) ensuring that the blocks include the most extensive spread visible to the naked eye; this may require the taking of oblique or eccentric blocks; see Figure 2.9(b).

The main disadvantage of cruciate blocking is that not all of the biopsy sample is embedded for histological examination; the 'corners' are usually returned to fixative and only embedded at a later stage if the original sections fail to provide clear evidence or otherwise of adequacy of excision. Unfortunately, accurate orientation of the 'corner' pieces is often impossible, and these subsequent paraffin blocks may give misleading information. For this reason we sometimes prefer the 'multilevel' blocking system illustrated in Figure 2.9(c), in which virtually the entire biopsy is embedded and examined histologically, with the potential for complete assessment of the lesion and its completeness of excision by multiple levels.

All pre-embedding trimming of skin biopsies should be carried out when the tissue has hardened after fixation; easier and more precise trimming of small samples can be achieved after complete dehydration in alcohol prior to wax embedding.

Punch biopsies

Punch biopsies are usually embedded entire with any trimming into a (presumed) small central lesion occurring during paraffin sectioning. If the lesion is a vesicle, macule or papule, several levels may need to be examined histologically until it is found. If the lesion is larger and occupies much of the biopsy, it is possible to trim off one-quarter to one-third of the sample under the dissecting microscope after it has been fixed in formalin; this is easier if the fixed specimen is hardened in increasing concentrations of alcohol, trimming being performed when the specimen has been in at least two changes of absolute alcohol. This is not usually possible when tissue processing is automatic, but with occasional specimens it is worth processing them by hand so that this can be carried out. In this way, the trimmed piece may be processed for some other investigation such as electron microscopy, and the bulk of the biopsy processed into paraffin or acrylic resin for light microscopy.

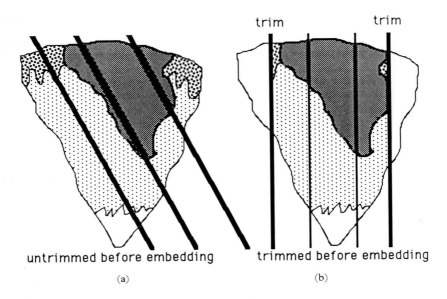

Fig. 2.8(a) and (b) Trimming of skin biopsies. (a) shows the obliquity of sections produced when there is no prior trimming. Trimming of one or both lateral edges, as in (b), produces vertical sections.

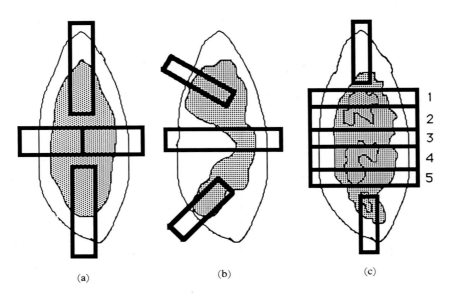

Fig 2.9(a), (b) and (c) Suggested block-taking patterns in excisional biopsies, particularly of tumours. (a) shows simple cruciate blocking to access completeness of excision of symmetrical lesions. (b) shows eccentric cruciate blocking of irregular tumours, and (c) shows a multilevel blocking scheme.

Table 2.1   Examples of histological methods used in dermatopathology

Method	Section	Uses
Haematoxylin and Eosin (H & E)	F, P, AR,	General architecture; cytology;
Periodic acid Schiff (PAS)	F, P, AR,	Basal lamina; fungi; mucin; glycogen
Elastic–van Gieson	F, P, AR,	Elastic fibres in dermis and skin vessels
Van Gieson	F, P, AR,	Collagen and muscle
Martius Scarlet Blue (MSB)	F, P,	Fibrin
Cresyl Fast Violet (CFV), Toluidine Blue	F, P, AR,	Mast cells
Congo/Sirius red	F, P, AR,	Amyloid
Methenamine silver	F, P, AR,	Fungi
Masson silver (e.g. Fontana)	F, P, AR,	Melanin
Perls Prussian Blue	F, P, AR,	Haemosiderin (iron)
Giemsa	F, P, AR,	Leishmania
Warthin-Starry	F, P,	Treponemes
Ziehl-Neelsen	F, P, AR,	Tubercle bacilli
Auramine-Rhodamine	F, P,	Tubercle bacilli
Wade-Fite	F, P, AR,	Leprosy bacilli
Oil Red O	F only	Lipids
Sudan Black	F, some P	Some lipids
Chloroacetate esterase	F, P, AR	Mast and myeloid cells
Alcian Blue	F, P, AR	Epithelial and stromal mucin

Note: The acrylic resin referred to in this table is glycol methacrylate; with other acrylics the methods may fail or need major modification before successful staining is obtained.
F = frozen section, P = paraffin section, AR = acrylic resin section

Curette biopsies

No orientation is possible; all fragments should be embedded, and histological sections prepared from a number of levels.

Shave biopsies

Since these are usually thin, and often curled over, they are best examined carefully under the dissecting microscope before the biopsy is trimmed prior to embedding, to ensure that the histological section is through the thickest part of the sample. Examination of a number of levels of the embedded tissue is also a wise precaution.

3.   Histology of normal skin

Introduction
The skin is a large and complex organ with a number of different functions, all of which, in one way and another, serve a protective purpose for the body as whole. The main specific functions are:
1.   Protection against external agents;
2.   Sensory;
3.   Thermoregulatory.
There are also a number of minor functions such as sercretory, excretory, vitamin D synthesis, endocrine functions and energy storage.

The skin as protection against external agents
The skin is the main interface between the body and the external environment, and is thus exposed to a variety of damaging stimuli, mechanical, physical, chemical and infective. The structure of the skin is such that it is resistant to most of the common damaging stimuli, and also has considerable recuperative and reparative potential should it sustain significant injury. The surface layer of *keratin* acts as a useful barrier to liquid agents because it is relatively water-proof. Constant turnover of epithelial cells in the *epidermis* continuously replenishes the surface keratin layer, and permits rapid regeneration of the protective epidermal layer should it be breached by injury. Certain areas of the skin, particularly the palms of the hands, pulps of the fingers, and soles of the feet, are constantly subjected to shearing stress which would tend to separate the epidermis from the underlying dermis (see shearing blisters, p. 62); this is minimized in these areas by the complex interdigitation of epidermis with dermis by a fully developed system of rete ridges (see Figs. 3.1(a), 3.17(a)). Elsewhere, in areas less subject to constant shearing forces, this rete ridge system is normally rudimentary or absent, but can reappear as an adaptive response to chronic trauma, e.g. in lichen simplex chronicus (see p. 42).

Skin may be exposed to various radiations, particularly U.V. light; the *melanin*, produced in epidermal *melanocytes*, absorbs much of this potentially damaging radiation. The effectiveness of this melanin screen can be assessed by the resistance of the negro skin to sunburn, even though the exposure during daylight hours is often severe and constant. Conversely, the susceptibility of white-skinned individuals to severe sunburn following quite short exposure to moderate amounts of sunlight is well-known; the adaptive response of increased melanin production and distribution increases the resistance of the white skin to subsequent UV light exposure and lessens the severity of acute skin damage.

The *dermis* is a tough, compact tissue with considerable resistance to penetration and physical damage; this is the result of it being formed of dense collagen bundles which are largely orientated parallel to the skin surface, and made mobile by the presence of intimately related elastic fibres. Dermal collagen is capable of being replenished by scattered resting fibrocytes, which are capable of activation into collagen-synthesizing fibroblasts if the need arises, as in the process of scar formation. Like the epidermis, the dermis is thickest and toughest in those areas most likely to be physically traumatized.

The skin as a sensory organ
The skin is well-supplied with sensory nerve endings which are sensitive to touch, heat and pain, thus providing an excellent protective mechanism, by warning the body of adverse environmental conditions which would be likely to cause tissue damage. Linked to an instant withdrawal mechanism mediated through the simple reflex arc, the system is effective in minimizing the risk of the body being damaged by the external environment.

The skin as a thermoregulatory organ
The skin has an unusually rich blood supply (see Fig. 3.1(b)) with many of the capillaries being situated near the tips of the dermal papillae, separated from the external environment only by a layer of epidermis a few cells in thickness. This provides a mechanism for heat exchange directly across the epidermis. Dilatation of the superficial capillaries, with increased flow through them, permits loss of heat to the environment in conditions of high body temperature. Constriction of capillaries, and reduced blood flow, reduces loss of heat from the body.

Sweat glands of *eccrine* type secrete a watery solution (sweat) onto the skin surface and the evaporation of this fluid has a pronounced cooling effect. Retention of body-heat is much more difficult to achieve, particularly now man has evolved from the extensive covering of the skin surface by thick body hair.

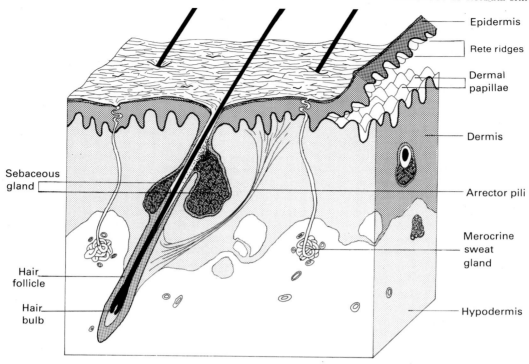

Epidermis

Rete ridges

Dermal papillae

Dermis

Sebaceous gland

Arrector pili

Merocrine sweat gland

Hair follicle

Hair bulb

Hypodermis

Fig. 3.1 (a)

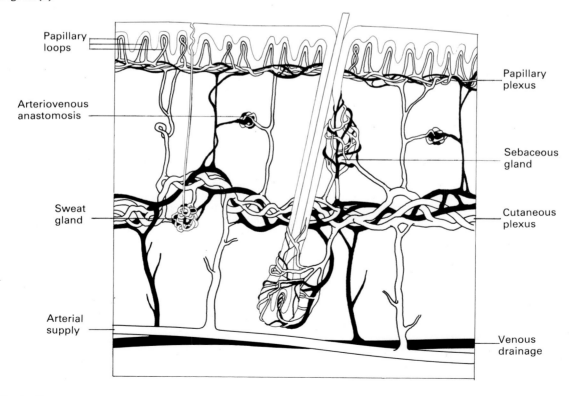

Papillary loops

Papillary plexus

Arteriovenous anastomosis

Sebaceous gland

Sweat gland

Cutaneous plexus

Arterial supply

Venous drainage

Fig. 3.1 (b)

Fig. 3.2(a)–(f) The epidermis (illustrations opposite)
The basic structure of the epidermis is that of a highly specialized, stratified squamous epithelium which, unlike its counterpart lining some of the body cavities, produces the fibrous proteinaceous material, *keratin*. Although there is considerable variation in the relative amounts of keratin and epithelium between skin from different anatomical sites, the structure of the epidermis conforms to a basic pattern.
There are four cell populations in the epidermis:

1. **Keratinocytes**;
2. **Melanocytes**;
3. **Langerhans cells**;
4. **Merkel cells**.

In terms of structural mass, the keratinocyte system is by far the most important population since these are the cells which account for and maintain the major mechanical and protective properties of skin.

Keratinocytes of the epidermis are in a constant state of production, maturation and exfoliation. In the non-diseased state the loss of cells by exfoliation is balanced by production of new cells by proliferation of stem cells in the epidermis. The turnover time from stem cell to exfoliation varies considerably between anatomical sites, but for the skin as a whole has been calculated at between 27 and 45 days.

As can be seen in Figure 3.2(a), which is a section of finger-tip skin, the keratinocytes of the epidermis can be divided into four morphologically different layers. In thin skin however, as in Figure 3.2(b) which is taken from the chest wall, these layers are much more difficult to identify. A fifth layer (stratum lucidum) is seen in the sole of the foot (see Fig. 3.17(a)).

Stratum basale **(i)**: The cells of this layer are cuboidal or columnar and form a single layer separated from the dermis by a basement membrane. In routine paraffin sections the basement membrane is usually impossible to identify unless a specific stain has been used, e.g. silver staining or PAS as in micrograph (f) in which the basement membrane is stained magenta (arrow). The cells of the basal layer (also called the stratum germinativum) serve as a source of stem cells for all keratinocytes and, like tissues containing stem cells elsewhere in the body, mitotic figures are frequently observed. Mitotic activity may also be seen in higher layers of the epidermis. The basal aspect of each stem keratinocyte or basal cell is highly irregular and bound to the basement membrane by numerous hemidesmosomes (see Fig. 3.3(a)). Like the cells of the adjacent stratum spinosum, small cytoplasmic projections extend across intercellular spaces to abut upon those of adjacent cells; these contact points are bound by desmosomes. Although the primary function of basal keratinocytes is eventual maturation into keratin, these cells also differentiate into the structures known as the skin appendages. In micrograph(e) the cuboidal or columnar nature of basal cells and irregular interdigitation with the dermis **(v)** is readily seen.

Stratum spinosum **(ii)**: Also known as the *prickle cell layer*, this consists of a variable number of layers of relatively large, polyhedral-shaped cells which are connected together by large numbers of opposed cytoplasmic projections ('prickles') bound by desmosomes. Prickles are well demonstrated in micrograph (d) which is a thin (1 µm) epoxy resin section stained by the Toluidine Blue method and discussed further in Figure 3.3b. The prominent nucleoli and cytoplasmic basophilia of the lower spinosum cells indicate active protein synthesis and indeed this is the zone in which basal cells start the process of differentiation into keratin. Nearer the surface the cytoplasmic basophilia is reduced. Fibrillar and amorphous proteins, the predominant synthetic products of these cells, aggregate to form intracellular fibrils known as *tonofibrils* (arrowed) which converge upon the desmosomes of the cytoplasmic prickles. The prickle cell layer is particularly deep in the thick skin shown in micrograph(a) and only two or three layers thick in the thin skin of micrograph (b). In the spinosal layer, in addition to the keratinocytes, there is a complex network of cytoplasmic dendritic processes from melanocytes and Langerhans cells.

Stratum granulosum **(iii)**: The characteristic feature of this layer, which is hardly visible in micrograph (b) showing thin skin, but two to three layers thick in micrograph (a), is the presence of dense basophilic granules which crowd the cytoplasm of the maturing keratinocytes which are by now becoming flatter and more elongated. The chemical nature of these so-called keratohyaline granules is distinct from that of the fibrous protein of the tonofibrils. The process of keratinization is thought to involve the combination of tonofibril and keratohyaline elements to form the mature keratin complex. The cells of the granular layer also synthesize membrane-bound glycophospholipid granules called keratinosomes which may form an intercellular cementing substance; see Figure 3.3(c). In the outermost aspect of the stratum granulosum, cell death occurs due to rupture of lysosomal membranes and the released enzymes may be important in the final process of keratinization.

Stratum corneum **(iv)**: This is seen as a wispy thin zone in micrographs (a) and (b), and as a thick layer in micrograph (c). The morphology and staining characteristics of this layer are strikingly different from the underlying layers. By this stage in the maturation of the keratinocyte, cell death has occurred, as indicated by the complete absence of viable intracellular organelles, as seen by both the light and electron microscope. The stratum corneum, or cornified layer, consists of layers of fused flattened vestiges of cells filled with mature keratin. In the deeper layers of the corneum the cells retain their desmosomal junctions and the intracellular keratin has an ordered pattern. Towards the surface, this ordered arrangement disintegrates, a process which precedes and may even initiate desquamation. Since the outer surface of the skin is constantly subject to mechanical forces, the loosely attached cornified cells of the outer stratum corneum are continuously lost into the outside environment.

Stratum lucidum: This layer is not shown in any of these micrographs. It is only reliably seen in sections of skin from sole of foot (see Fig. 3.17(a)) and occasionally in skin from the palm of the hand. When it does occur it consists of several layers of closely packed, flattened, anucleate cells which gives it a homogeneous, hyaline appearance in histological section. Its functional significance is unknown and may merely represent a compressed transitional zone between the granular layer and the cornified layer.

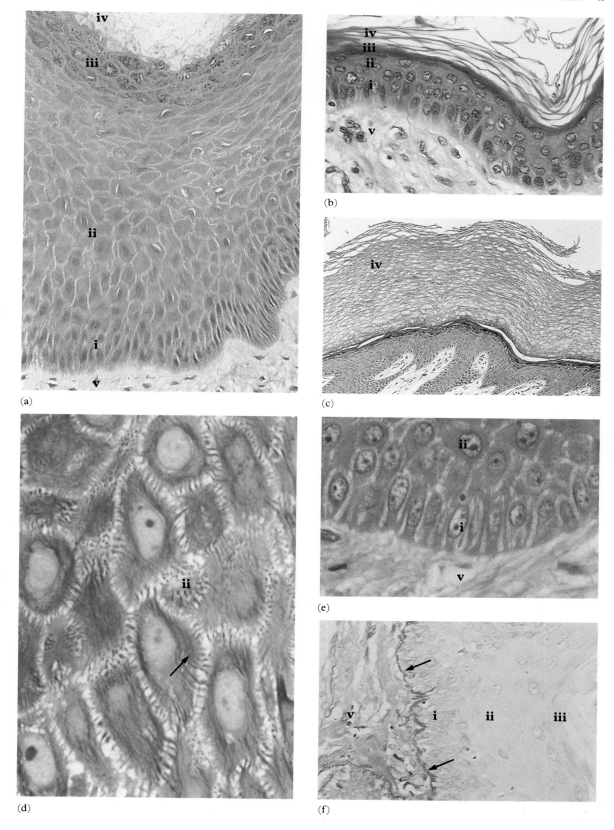

(a)

(b)

(c)

(d)

(e)

(f)

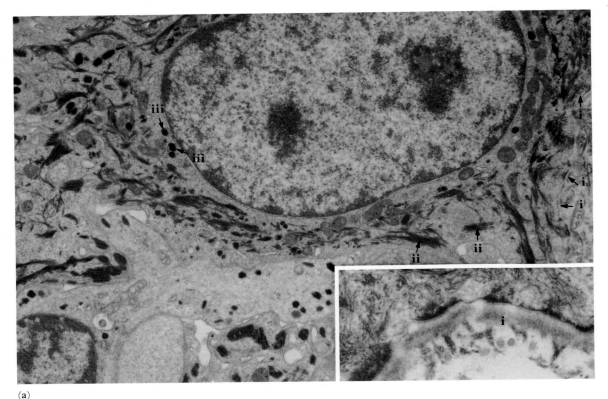

(a)

Fig. 3.3(a), (b) & (c) Ultrastructure of Epidermal Keratinocytes

(a) **Basal keratinocyte**: this electron micrograph shows a typical basal cell. It is roughly columnar in shape. Its lower border is attached to the slightly convoluted basal lamina **(i)** by hemidesmosomes (see inset), its lateral borders to adjacent basal cells by sparse desmosomes, and to the overlying keratinocytes of the prickle cell layer (stratum spinosum) by abundant well-formed desmosomes; see Figure 3.3(b) inset. The cell has a roughly ovoid nucleus, orientated in the long axis of the cell, with prominent chromatin networks and nucleoli; the cytoplasm is packed with organelles, including ribosomes, mitochondria and some tonofibrils. Ribosomes are particularly numerous and are responsible for the slight basophilia which the basal cell shows on routine H & E staining (this is due to the high RNA content); they are an indicator of active protein synthesis. Tonofibrils are present **(ii)**, but are much less numerous than in overlying spinous keratinocytes; see (b). In people with pigmented skins, basal keratinocytes also contain melanin granules **(iii)** transferred to them from the dendritic processes of adjacent melanocytes which insinuate themselves between the keratinocytes. Lysosomes are present in basal keratinocytes and are particularly prominent, in the form of phagolysosomes, in skin which has been exposed to injury, e.g. heat or light exposure; some phagolysosomes contain digested melanin.

(b) **Spinous Keratinocyte ('prickle cell')**: in the lower epidermis, near the basal keratinocyte layer, these cells are polygonal and are attached to each other by well-formed desmosomes (see inset). As they near the surface they become more flattened. Apart from their connecting desmosomes, keratinocytes in the upper layers of the stratum spinosum are characterized by the presence of

broad dense masses of cytoplasmic tonofibrils, some of which tail into the desmosomes; ribosomes are fewer than in basal keratinocytes and lower spinous cells, and the combination of this and increased numbers of proteinaceous tonofibrils gives the cytoplasm of these upper cells their slightly eosinophilic staining characteristics on H & E staining. Note the numerous dendritic processes of melanocytes **(iv)** and Langerhans cells **(v)** between the cytoplasmic 'prickles' which link adjacent keratinocytes (see also Fig. 3.9).

(c) **Granular keratinocyte**: as they near the surface the flattened spinous keratinocytes develop round or oval granules with a variably complex lamellar structure, called keratinosomes or 'Odland bodies' (see inset). These are first seen close to the Golgi body, but then extend into the cytoplasm where they partially disrupt and their glycophospholipid component is extruded into the intercellular spaces. This glycophospholipid acts as 'glue', holding together the cellular and keratin components of the stratum corneum, and providing a hydrophobic barrier in the superficial skin layer, rendering it non-wettable. At the same time, dense osmiophilic bodies (keratohyaline granules: **(vi)**) appear in the cytoplasm of the flattened keratinocytes and gradually dominate the cytoplasm, with other cytoplasmic organelles and the nucleus disappearing. The keratohyaline and the cytoplasmic tonofibrils survive to become the keratin layer; the precise nature of keratohyaline is not known but it is proteinaceous and rich in sulphur-containing amino-acids such as cystine.

The deeper layers of the stratum corneum **(vii)** therefore consist of flattened cells which are largely sheets of keratohyaline intermingled with tonofibrils bounded by a cell membrane and include nuclear and cytoplasmic remnants. The superficial layers are anucleate.

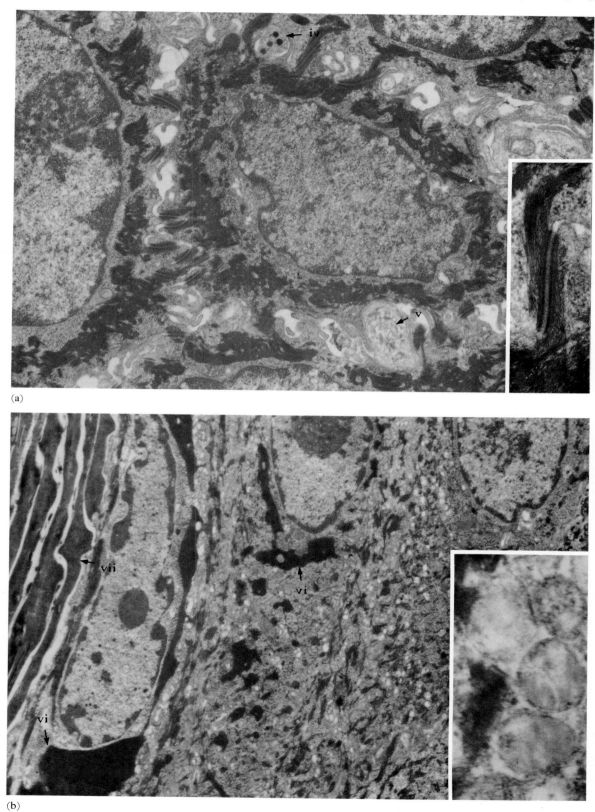

(a)

(b)

Non-keratinizing cells of the epidermis

Melanocytes
These are the cells responsible for skin pigmentation and are of neuro-ectodermal origin. Melanocytes are dendritic cells most commonly found scattered amongst basal keratinocytes, and are discussed further in Figures 3.4, 3.5 and 3.6.

Langerhans cells
These are also dendritic cells found both amongst the basal layers of epidermis and in the stratum spinosum. In routine preparations they appear as pale-stained cells with an indented nucleus (see Figures 3.7, 3.8 and 3.9). Langerhans cells are thought to be derived from bone-marrow and represent part of a reticulo-epithelial system which is involved in antigen-handling in epithelial surfaces, in this case the epidermis. Unlike the stem cell populations of the epidermis, Langerhans cells are able to migrate to lymphoid tissues and stimulate the production of specific lymphocyte populations in response to a specific antigen.

Merkel cells
These are also thought to be embryologically derived from neural crest tissue and are a population of cells scattered throughout the basal epidermis. They occur most commonly in association with intra-epithelial nerve endings and are thought to be associated with a sensory function. Merkel cells have a characteristic ultrastructural appearance, containing fewer cytoplasmic filaments than surrounding keratinocytes and having a number of electron-dense granules of neuro-endocrine type. They cannot be identified with certainty in light microscope sections without the use of specific histochemical and immunohistochemical staining techniques. There is some evidence that they may be a component of the diffuse neuro-endocrine system.

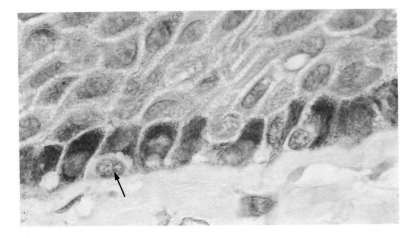

Fig. 3.4 Negroid abdominal skin
The colour of human skin is not only dependent on the presence of the pigment melanin but also on yellowish carotene pigments in subcutaneous fat, the concentration and state of oxygenation of blood in its blood vessels and the presence of chromogens in blood such as bile pigments. The presence and amount of melanin is the most important variable between parts of the body, between individuals of the same race and between members of different races. In comparison with Figure 3.2(e), this micrograph demonstrates the relative abundance of darkly pigmented melanin in the basal layers of negroid skin. Melanocytes themselves may be difficult to identify in routine H & E-stained preparations of negro skin. Note also that some of the cells of the stratum spinosum contain significant amounts of melanin. The ratio of melanocytes to basal cells is from one in five to one in ten, being highest in the face and external genitalia. There is relatively no inter-racial difference in the number of melanocytes, colour differences between races being due to the amount of melanin produced.

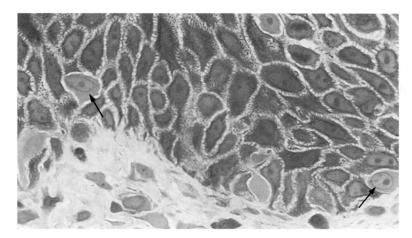

Fig. 3.5. Melanocyte-Tol Blue Resin section

This micrograph illustrates the typical light microscope appearance of melanocytes in Caucasian skin. Identification of these cells is facilitated by the use of resin-embedding and thin sectioning. Melanocytes (arrow) are readily differentiated from adjacent basal cells: they have large ovoid nuclei with dispersed chromatin and abundant perinuclear cytoplasm which extends into long cytoplasmic extensions between local keratinocytes. In routine H & E paraffin sections melanocytes also have clear cytoplasm, but their dendritic processes are more difficult to see.

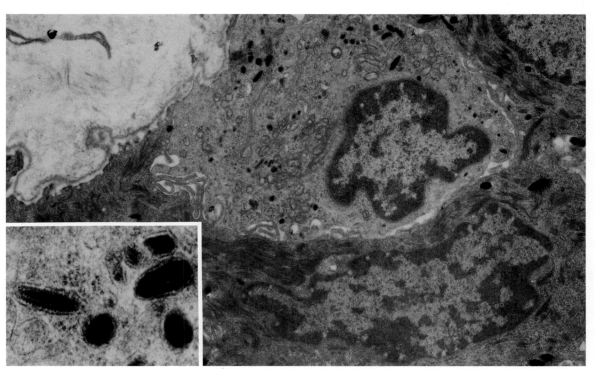

Fig. 3.6. Melanocyte: ultrastructural features

The melanocyte seen in this electron micrograph can be distinguished from surrounding keratinocytes by its paler cytoplasm, absence of tonofilaments and desmosomes, and its content of membrane-bound premelanosomes and melanosomes. Premelanosomes are ovoid cytoplasmic bodies showing characteristic striations (see inset); melanin is synthesized within them to form melanosomes. Melanin synthesis involves the conversion of the amino acid tyrosine via DOPA to melanin, which is then linked to a protein. With the increasing deposition of melanin in the premelanosomes, the striated pattern is obscured and the organelle becomes more rounded. The long dendritic processes of melanocytes ramify between basal and spinous keratinocytes but do not appear to establish cell junctions

with them. Nevertheless, the melanosomes containing melanin are transferred to surrounding keratinocytes by a process which is not understood. Hence, the pigmented cells of the epidermis consist of both melanocytes and keratinocytes. Paradoxically, keratinocytes often contain much more melanin than melanocytes. The size, shape and rate of melanosome production varies greatly between individuals and racial groups. In blond and red-haired people melanin is biochemically different. The ultraviolet component of sunlight not only stimulates melanin synthesis but also darkens previously synthesized melanin. In addition, melanin synthesis is stimulated by the pituitary hormome MSH, although the physiological significance of this in humans is not well understood.

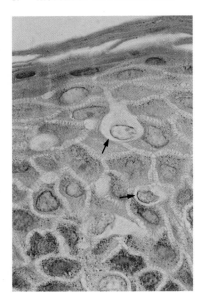

Fig. 3.7. Langerhans cell

These cells are found scattered amongst the stratum basale and stratum spinosum, are encountered relatively infrequently and have a characteristic pale-stained dendritic cytoplasm with an indented nucleus. They are not connected to adjacent cells by prickles and do not contain melanin. Positive identification of Langerhans cells can be supported by electron microscopical identification of Birbeck granules and the immunocytochemical demonstration of T6 reactivity (see Figs. 3.8 and 3.9).

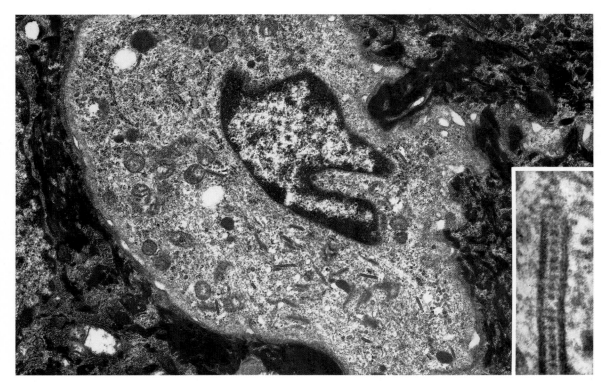

Fig. 3.8 Langerhans cell: transmission E.M.

This micrograph of part of a Langerhans cell shows some of its characteristic features. Unlike surrounding keratinocytes it contains no tonofilaments and is not attached via desmosomes−an observation consistent with its migratory role in antigen processing and collaboration with distant lymphoid tissues. The distinctive ultrastructural feature of this cell is the presence of Birbeck granules (see inset), most of which are rod-like structures with periodic cross

striations. Occasionally, these rods have a terminal dilatation, as in the inset, giving rise to a 'tennis racquet' conformation and hence the term *tennis racquet granule*. These organelles have no known functional significance but can be used as a cell marker for the diagnosis of the Langerhans cell-derived tumour histiocytosis X (see Fig. 22.12). The role of these cells in normal physiological processes remains to be fully elucidated.

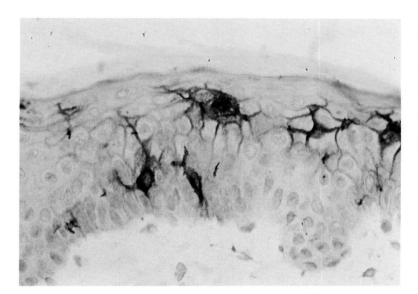

Fig. 3.9. Langerhans cell: immunocytochemical reactivity
This micrograph shows epidermis which is abnormal due to chronic atopic dermatitis; it contains increased numbers of Langerhans cells, demonstrated here by the immunocytochemical method for T6 antigen. With this technique the Langerhans cells appear as brown spidery cells, the legs of the spider representing the dendritic processes which ramify between keratinocytes.

Skin appendages

In various parts of the skin surface the epidermis forms highly specialized structures which are all derived from multipotential basal keratinocytes. These so-called skin appendages include hair follicles, sebaceous glands and sweat glands. Most sebaceous glands discharge their oily content, sebum, onto the skin surface via ducts into hair follicles; the combination of hair follicle and sebaceous gland is termed a *pilosebaceous unit*. In some sites, notably nipple, external genitalia, lips and the eyelid, sebaceous glands discharge their secretions directly onto the surface. The sweat glands are divided into two types depending on their mode of secretion: the most common type is the *eccrine* or *merocrine* sweat gland which is widely distributed throughout the skin surface except on the glans penis, clitoris, lips, labia minora and under the nails. These glands are largely involved in thermoregulation. *Apocrine* sweat glands are found mainly in the axilla, peri-anal region and associated with the external genitalia. Unlike eccrine sweat glands, the apocrine glands begin to function only at puberty and are thought to be involved largely in the production of sexually attractive odours. Nails are highly specialised products of keratinisation and are found only on the dorsal aspect of the ends of the fingers and toes.

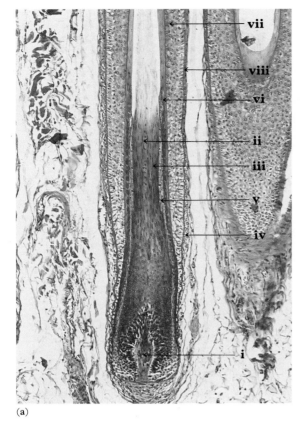

(a)

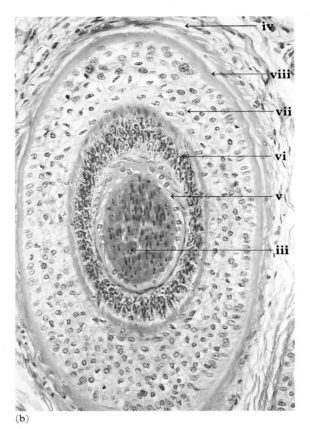

(b)

Fig. 3.10(a) & (b). Hair follicle LS and TS

The hair follicle is a tubular structure consisting of five concentric layers of epithelial cells. At the base, there is a bulbous expansion, the hair bulb, enclosing the dermal papilla **(i)**. As they are pushed towards the skin surface from the hair bulb, the inner three layers undergo keratinization to form the hair shaft, whilst the outer two layers form an epithelial sheath. At the hair bulb, all the layers merge to become indistinguishable from one another.

During active hair growth, the epithelial cells surrounding the dermal papilla proliferate to form the innermost four layers of the follicle whilst the outermost layer merely represents a downward continuation of the stratum germinativum of the surface epithelium. The whole epithelial mass surrounding the dermal papilla constitutes the hair root.

The cells of the innermost layer of the follicle undergo moderate keratinization to form the medulla **(ii)** or core of the hair shaft; the medullary layer is often not distinguishable in fine hairs. The medulla is surrounded by a broad, highly keratinized layer, the cortex **(iii)** which forms the bulk of the hair. The third cell layer of the follicle undergoes keratinization to form a hard, thin cuticle **(v)** on the surface of the hair. The cuticle consists of overlapping keratin plates, an arrangement which is said to prevent matting of the hair.

The fourth layer of the follicle constitutes the internal root sheath **(vi)**; the cells of this layer become only lightly keratinized and disintegrate at the level of the sebaceous gland ducts leaving a space into which sebum is secreted around the maturing hair. The outermost layer, the external root sheath **(vii)**, does not take part in hair formation: this layer is separated from the sheath of connective tissue **(iv)** surrounding the follicle by a thick, specialized basement membrane known as the glassy membrane **(viii)**.

In the growing follicle, the large active melanocytes are scattered amongst the proliferating cells forming the cortex of the hair shaft, thereby determining hair colour. In micrograph (b) which is a slightly oblique transverse section through the lower part of a hair follicle, the broad external root sheath **(vii)** is separated from the connective tissue sheath **(iv)** by the glassy membrane **(viii)**. Passing inwards, the internal root sheath is recognized by its content of eosinophilic (keratohyaline) granules; the outermost cells of the internal root sheath have a more homogeneous appearance. Deep to the internal root sheath is the thin pale-stained cuticle layer **(v)** which surrounds the strongly stained cortex **(iii)**. A medulla is not present in this specimen.

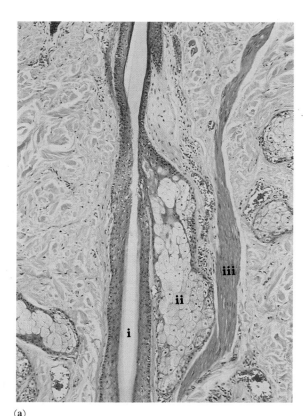

(a)

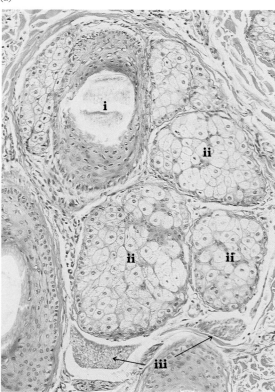

(b)

Fig. 3.11(a) & (b). Sebaceous gland

These micrographs illustrate the relationships of a sebaceous gland **(ii)** and an arrector pili muscle **(iii)** to a hair follicle **(i)**, both in longitudinal (a) and transverse (b) section. At a point about one-third of its length from the surface, each hair follicle is surrounded by one or more sebaceous glands which discharge their secretions onto the hair shaft and thence onto the skin surface. Sebaceous glands lie within the connective tissue sheath surrounding the hair follicle and the glandular epithelium represents an outgrowth of the external root sheath.

The arrector pili muscle of each follicle consists of a bundle of smooth muscle fibres. The muscle inserts at one end into the connective tissue sheath of the follicle, at a point below the sebaceous glands, and at the other end into the dermal papillary area beneath the epidermis. Each hair follicle and its associated arrector pili muscle and sebaceous glands is known as a pilosebaceous unit.

Each sebaceous gland has a branched acinar form, the acini converging upon a short duct which empties into the hair follicle beside the maturing hair. Each acinus consists of a mass of rounded cells which are packed with lipid-filled vacuoles; during tissue preparation the lipid is largely removed, with the result that the cytoplasm of these cells is poorly stained. Towards the duct, the lipid content of the acinar cells increases greatly and the distended cells degenerate, so releasing their contents, sebum, into the ducts by the process known as holocrine secretion. Cells lost by holocrine secretion are replaced by mitosis in the basal layer of the acinus by proliferation of basal cells. Like apocrine sweat glands, sebaceous glands are under hormone control and proliferate at puberty.

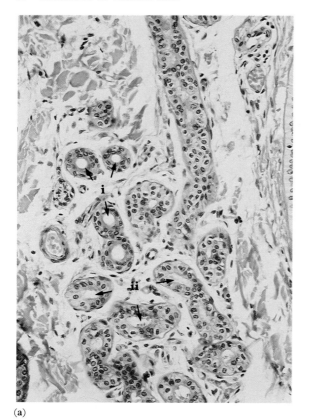

(a)

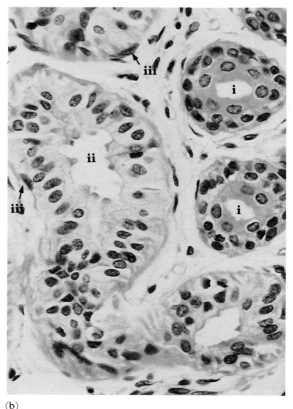

(b)

Fig. 3.12(a) & (b). Eccrine (merocrine) sweat gland
Eccrine sweat glands are distributed in the skin of most
parts of the body. These glands secrete a watery fluid
(hypotonic with respect to plasma) the evaporation of which
plays an important role in thermoregulation. Sweat contains
significant quantities of sodium and chloride ions, some
other ions, urea and small molecular weight metabolites;
thus sweating may be considered as a minor mode of
excretion.

Eccrine sweat glands are unbranched, tubular glands,
the secretory portion of which forms a compact coil deep in
the dermis. In histological section, the glands appear as a
mass of tubules cut in various planes; secretory portions are
interspersed with sections of the first part of the excretory
duct. The secretory portion **(ii)** consists of a single layer of
large cuboidal or columnar cells, whereas the excretory duct
(i) is lined by two layers of smaller cuboidal cells. The
surrounding dermal connective tissue contains a rich
capillary plexus.

At higher magnification in (b), the secretory portions
(ii) of eccrine sweat glands are seen to be mainly composed

of pale-stained, pyramidal-shaped cells which rest on a
prominent basement membrane. These cells are believed to
pump sodium ions into the gland lumen; this is followed by
passive diffusion of water. A second, darkly-stained cell
type which is difficult to identify with light microscopy is
described; this cell type has ultrastructural features typical
of protein-secreting cells. The dark cells are believed to
secrete a glycoprotein although the content of such in sweat
is very low. Myoepithelial cells **(iii)** form a discontinuous
layer between the secretory cells and the basement
membrane; contraction of these cells expels sweat into the
excretory ducts.

Sections of the excretory duct **(i)** are readily
distinguishable from sections of the secretory portion. The
excretory duct has a narrower lumen, a double layer of small
cuboidal cells, no underlying myoepithelial cells and a
characteristically eosinophilic luminal aspect which may
result from adsorption of the glycoprotein product of the
dark secretory cells. The duct epithelium is thought to
reabsorb sodium ions from the basic secretion thus making
it hypotonic with respect to plasma.

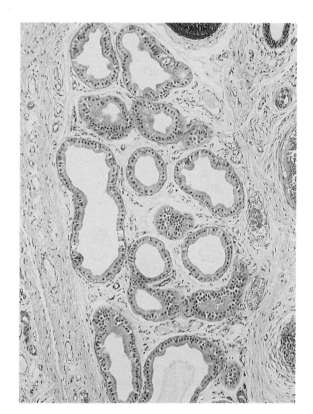

Fig. 3.13. Apocrine sweat gland

Apocrine sweat glands are mainly confined to the axillae and genital regions where they produce a viscid, milky secretion which becomes odorous after the action of skin commensal bacteria.

Apocrine sweat glands are large glands which always secrete into an adjacent hair follicle via a duct which is histologically similar to that of eccrine sweat glands. The secretory portion of the gland is of the coiled, tubular type with a widely dilated lumen. The secretory cells are usually low cuboidal and have an eosinophilic cytoplasm. The budding appearance of the apical cytoplasm of some cells gave rise to the belief that the mode of secretion was of the apocrine type but recent evidence suggests that this appearance may be due to a fixation artefact and that the original interpretations were erroneous. Apocrine sweat glands secrete by apocrine, mesocrine and holocrine processes. Like eccrine sweat glands, apocrine glands have a discontinuous layer of myoepithelial cells between the base of the secretory cells and the prominent basement membrane.

Apocrine sweat glands do not become functional until puberty and in women undergo cyclical changes under the influence of the hormones of the menstrual cycle. The so-called *ceruminous glands* of the external auditory meatus are a specific type of apocrine sweat gland and their secretions mixed with locally produced sebum forms the substance known as earwax.

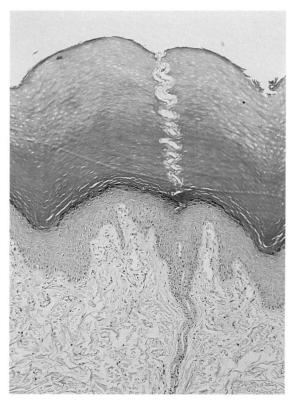

Fig. 3.14. Eccrine sweat duct emerging through thick skin

The duct of an eccrine sweat gland is coiled at its origin from the sweat gland, but then runs vertically straight up to the dermo-epidermal junction. It then becomes spiral again in its passage to the exterior through the epidermis; this intra-epidermal component is known as the acrosyrinx or acrosyringium, a term rarely used except in the context of the nomenclature of benign tumours believed to be derived from this part of the sweat duct. The intra-epidermal part is best seen in thick skin, as in the sole of the foot in this micrograph; note that the spiral pattern is reflected in the thick stratum corneum.

The dermis and hypodermis

In all areas of the skin surface the epidermis is supported by a concective tissue layer called the dermis. This layer not only varies in thickness from site to site, but also in its constituent parts. The interface between epidermis and dermis is also highly variable in conformation; in thin skin it is relatively smooth whereas in thick skin it is highly ridged.

The connective tissue framework of the dermis is largely collagenous but variable amounts of elastic fibres and reticulin fibres are also embedded in an amorphous ground substance. With advancing age there is a relative loss of elasticity as individual fibres become thickened and hyalinized. The cellular components of the dermis consist of macrophages, mast cells, fibroblasts, migrating cells of the leucocyte series, and occasional melanocytes and adipocytes. The dermis offers support for blood vessels, lymphatics and nerves as well as the skin appendages. In some sites, e.g. the nipple and scrotum, the dermis contains bundles of smooth muscle fibres and in the face, the striated muscle fibres of the muscles of facial expression terminate in the dermis.

Histologically, two discrete areas of the dermis can be recognized; beneath the epidermis there is a relatively loose arrangement of connective tissue called the *papillary dermis* which has thin collagen fibres, many small blood vessels and a relatively large amount of ground substance. This area of the dermis is thrown up into dermal papillae which interdigitate with downward projections of the epidermis and in the finger-tips, forms the structural basis of fingerprints. Deep to this is the so-called *reticular dermis* which has a denser pattern of coarse collagen fibres and contains fewer capillaries and exogenous cell populations. Strands of the reticular dermis project through the hypodermis and fuse with underlying fascial or periosteal layers.

The dermis in general contains at any one time around 50% of the circulating blood volume. There are numerous arteriovenous shunts and blood may be rapidly diverted to the upper dermis for the purposes of cooling as part of the process of thermoregulation. Not only are the epidermis and the skin appendages totally dependent for oxygen and nutrition on diffusion of these substances from the dermis, but the dermis exerts a developmentally inductive effect in terms of control of cellular proliferation and differentiation.

In functional terms the dermis protects and supports the epidermis, anchors the epidermis to underlying tissues, provides a barrier to infections and is the major element of the skin's resistance to mechanical trauma. It is also the major site of wound healing after the skin surface has been breached or torn.

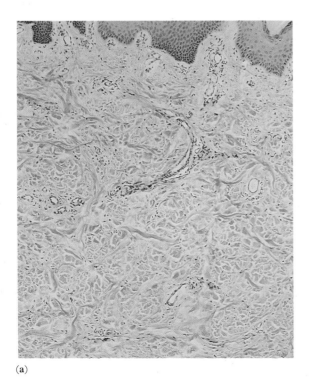

(a)

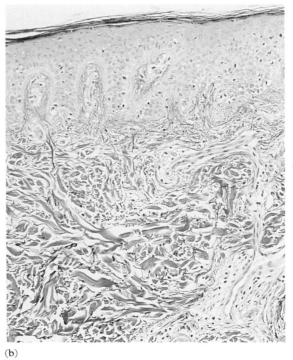

(b)

Fig. 3.15(a) and (b). Text opposite

Fig. 3.15 Dermis: (a) H & E and (b) EVG (illustrations opposite)

Note the pale-staining papillary dermis and the darker-staining reticular dermis. In the latter the collagen fibres form thick broad bundles, mainly running parallel to the surface interspersed with thick elastic fibres (black) in (b). In the papillary dermis the collagen and elastic fibres are fine and mainly haphazardly arranged, although when the papillae are prominent, both fibre types are perpendicular. Collagen and elastic fibres are embedded in a mucinous ground substance containing acid mucopolysaccharides, including dermatan sulphate, chondroitin sulphate and hyaluronic acid. This ground substance is normally most abundant in the papillary dermis and around skin appendages, but cannot be seen in a routine H & E-stained section; a staining method for acid mucopolysaccharides, such as Alcian Blue, is required.

Collagen and elastin fibres, and ground substance, are produced by spindle-celled fibroblasts, the most frequent and important cell in the normal dermis. Mast cells are present scattered sparsely through the dermis between collagen fibres but tend to be concentrated around blood vessels. Other cells frequently present in the dermis are wandering cells such as macrophages and lymphocytes; normally scanty, these cells are present in increased numbers in all inflammatory skin conditions.

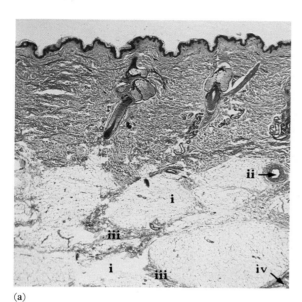

(a)

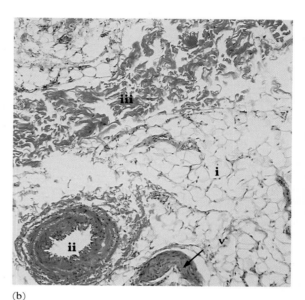

(b)

Fig. 3.16, Hypodermis (subcutis) (a) LP abdominal skin (b) HP

The zone of tissue beneath the reticular dermis and the underlying deep fascia, aponeurosis or periosteum is termed the *hypodermis* or subcutis. This is a layer of loose connective tissue with not only a highly variable and indistinct interface with the overlying dermis but also of widely variable thickness and composition. The collagenous fibres of the hypodermis are continuous with those of the dermis and mainly run parallel to the surface of the skin as in this micrograph. Where the skin is closely applied to underlying structures the collagenous component of the hypodermis is prolific, e.g. in solar and palmar skin. Depending on the site and the nutritional status of the individual the hypodermis may contain enormous amounts of adipose tissue. In Western society it is not uncommon for the hypodermis of abdominal skin to contain a 3 or 4 cm layer of adipose tissue; in this situation the hypodermis is termed anatomically the *panniculus adiposus*. On the other hand, the hypodermis of the eyelids and penis does not normally possess fat cells. The hypodermis of the skin overlying the face and neck contains sheets of skeletal muscle of the facial expression and platysma muscle, and in this situation the layer is called the *panniculus carnosus* which is a vestige of the flank muscles of lower mammals, in particular the horse.

In addition to its metabolic role in fat storage the hypodermis acts as a cushion against external trauma and provides attachment for the overlying skin to the tissues underneath. Almost without exception the hypodermis conducts and contains the large blood vessels and nerves which serve the skin, as in this micrograph. In some areas of skin specialized for sensory reception such as finger tip and external genitalia, the hypodermis also contains large encapsulated nerve endings called *Pacinian corpuscles* which are sensory organs responsive to pressure, coarse touch, vibration and tension. This micrograph, showing a section of hypodermis from abdomen shows adipose tissue (i), large blood vessels (ii), septae of collagenous connective tissue (iii), underlying deep fascia (iv), and occasional nerve trunks (v).

Fig. 3.17(a)–(d) Skin as a protective organ

The primary function of skin as a protective organ is not only manifest by the structure of every one of its constituent parts, but is also epitomized by its exhibition of regional variations in structure. In sites which are coninuously subject to frictional stresses and shearing forces, such as the sole of the foot and the palm of the hand, the epidermis can be seen to have attained its greatest development. In micrograph (a), a section from the sole of foot, there is an unusually thick stratum corneum while the curious stratum lucidum (arrow) is also clearly visible. This thick stratum corneum is able to withstand considerable frictional forces. In order to maintain such a thick cornified layer there is a correspondingly thick living epidermis (stratum basale plus spinosum plus granulosum) which is also evident from this micrograph. Finally, the interface between the epidermis and dermis is seen to be almost corrugated in configuration, an arrangement which permits significant resistance to shearing forces.

Another constituent of skin, the sebaceous gland, has a protective function, i.e. the production of the oily secretion, sebum. It is thought that sebum adds the final waterproofing property to the surface of the cornified layer although the odour of sebaceous secretion may be an important feature of sexual attraction. This latter theory is derived from the observation that sebaceous gland activity is hormonally dependent and that sebaceous glands in general are known to proliferate and develop at the onset of puberty. Micrograph (b) shows a longitudinal section through a pilosebaceous unit with a sebaceous gland acinus emptying into a hair follicle. The dermal connective tissue is seen to be condensed around the whole structure to form a pseudocapsule.

A regional variation in skin structure which is particularly adapted for the protective function occurs on the dorsal surface of the fingers and toes and takes the form of the nails. In micrograph (c), each nail (ii) is a dense, keratinized plate which rests on a stratified squamous epithelium called the nail bed. The proximal end of the nail, the nail root (vi), and the underlying nail bed extend deeply into the dermis to lie in close apposition to the distal interphalangeal joint, and the dermis beneath the nail plate is firmly attached to the periosteum of the distal phalanx (iv).

Nail growth occurs by proliferation and differentiation of the epithelium surrounding the nail root, and the nail plate slides distally over the rest of the nail bed which does not actively contribute to nail growth. Reflecting its proliferative activity, the epithelium beneath the nail root is thicker than that of the rest of the nail bed and exhibits pronounced epidermal ridges as seen in micrograph (d).

The skin overlying the root of the nail is known as the nail fold (v) and its highly keratinized free edge is known as the eponychium (i). The skin beneath the free end of the nail is known as the hyponychium (iii).

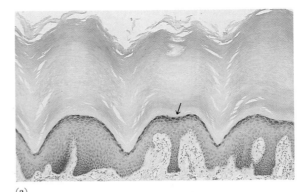

(a)

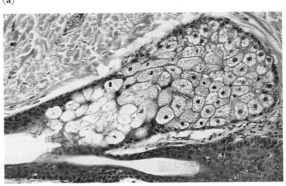

(b)

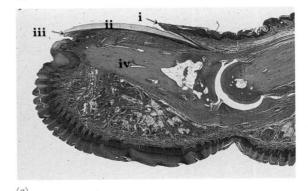

(c)

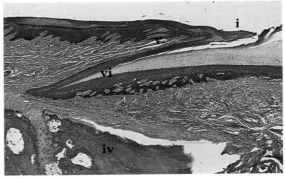

(d)

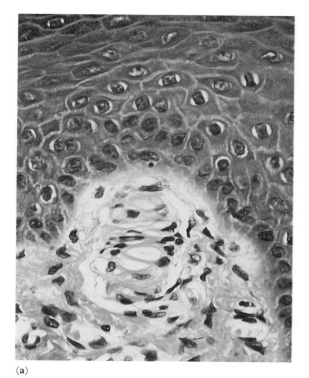

(a)

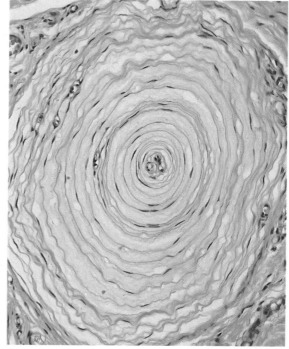

(b)

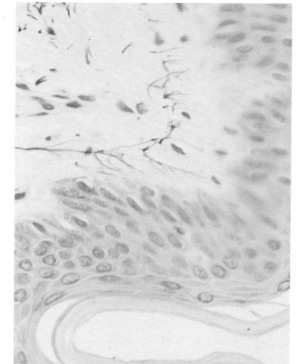

(c)

Fig. 3.18(a), (b) & (c). Skin as a sensory organ

The skin is the largest sensory organ in the body and constantly receives and mediates the flow of information between the external environment and the internal environment. The sensory receptors of skin are sensitive to heat, cold, light touch, deep touch, pain and vibration; they are particularly prominent and concentrated in the palmar and plantar surfaces, the genitalia and the lips. The sensory receptors of the skin are either encapsulated organs (Meissner's corpuscles and Pacinian corpuscles) or naked nerve endings. Micrograph (a) shows a Meissner's corpuscle in its characteristic location in a dermal papilla immediately beneath the epidermis; this receptor is oval in shape and consists of a delicate connective tissue capsule surrounding a mass of plump, oval cells (primary sensory nerves) arranged transversely. Non-myelinated branches of large myelinated sensory fibres ramify throughout the corpuscle. These corpuscles are involved in the reception of light touch sensation.

Micrograph (b) shows a Pacinian corpuscle deep in the hypodermis of finger tip skin; these large, encapsulated sensory organs are sensitive to coarse touch, vibration and tension, and are found in many sites throughout the body. In section, Pacinian corpuscles have the appearance of a cut onion; they consist of a delicate connective tissue capsule enclosing many lamellae of flattened cells separated by interstitial fluid. In the centre, the lamellae are closely packed around a core which contains a single large unmyelinated nerve fibre which becomes myelinated as it leaves the corpuscle.

Micrograph (c) shows a single unencapsulated nerve ending which terminates in the epidermis and, although not obvious in this section, is probably related to a Merkel cell. Such nerve endings are not visible in routine sections of skin and require specialized silver impregnation techniques for their demonstration as in this micrograph.

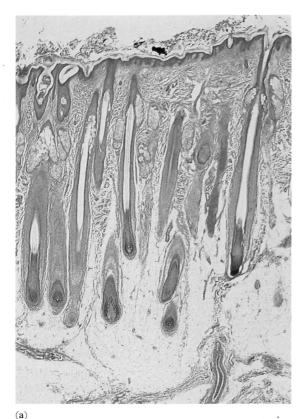

(a)

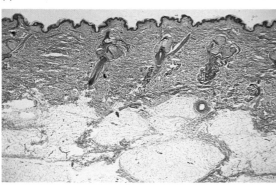

(b)

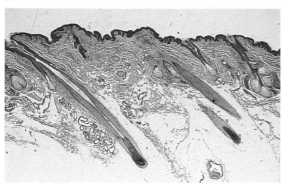

(c)

Fig. 3.19. Hairy skin (a) Scalp skin (b) Abdominal skin & (c) Pubic skin

These micrographs illustrates three extremes of structure in hairy skin.

As seen in micrograph (a), the skin of the scalp is robust due to a thick, densely collagenous dermis, and the hair follicles are numerous and closely packed. In fair-haired people, the follicles are fewer in number and somewhat smaller in size, producing finer hair. The follicles of the scalp are particularly long and have more numerous sebaceous glands than those of other areas. Note the arrector pili muscles extending from the base of the follicles towards the upper dermis. Merocrine sweat glands are numerous, though less prominent than in the skin of the trunk and limbs due to the profusion of other appendages.

Micrograph (b) illustrates the typical histological appearance of the skin which covers most of the body. The hair follicles and associated sebaceous glands are sparse and merocrine sweat glands are relatively abundant. The hair follicles are shorter and the hairs produced are finer.

The skin of the axillae and pubic region, shown in micrograph (c), contains a moderate density of hair follicles which, unlike those of the scalp, tend to be oriented obliquely to the skin surface and are often curved rather than straight, causing the hairs to be curled. Apocrine sweat glands are a common feature of this type of skin and are seen typically associated with hair follicles into which they discharge their secretions.

4. Illustrated glossary of dermatopathological terms

Introduction

Most dermatological conditions were originally described at a time when there was little knowledge of the aetiology or pathogenesis of the diseases, so the emphasis was on description, often with an attached eponym. Unfortunately, the position is slow to alter, but increasingly we are able to give skin conditions simpler and more informative names, e.g. linear IgA disease, which at least provide some clue to the underlying abnormality at the tissue level, if not the acutal cause. Sadly, even where the aetiology and pathogenesis of an eruption is known, there remains a regrettable tendency to name newly recognized conditions in the old manner; for the sake of clarity and understanding this should be resisted.

The vocabulary of terms used to describe some of the histological changes seen in skin lesions are peculiar to dermatopathology and can be confusing to trainee dermatologists and to pathologists inexperienced in the histological examination of abnormal skin. This chapter is an illustrated guide to some of the more commonly encountered terms specific to dermatopathology, as well as a few terms used in general pathology which experience has shown us to confuse dermatologists; many examples of the terms defined and illustrated here will be found scattered throughout this book.

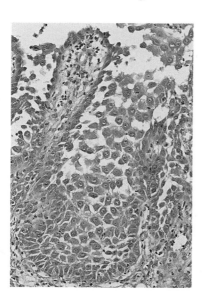

Fig. 4.1 Acantholysis

This is the name given to the process in which there is loss of adhesion and, subsequently, contact between epidermal cells, such that the cells separate one from the other with breakdown of desmosomal junctions and increase in the intercellular space. Eventually the intercellular space becomes large and fluid-filled, the separated acantholytic cells tending to become rounded off and floating singly or in small clumps within a variably sized bulla (see Figs. 8.4, 8.6). The precise causes of acantholysis are not known, but in pemphigus vulgaris, dissolution of the epidermal cell glycocalyx is an early pre-acantholytic feature, whereas acantholysis is frequently observed as a probable secondary phenomenon to epidermal cell necrosis in viral vesicles (see Fig. 10.1) and other conditions in which epidermal cells are damaged ('secondary acantholysis'). Examples of acantholysis in the epidermis are illustrated in Figures 17.5, 17.6.

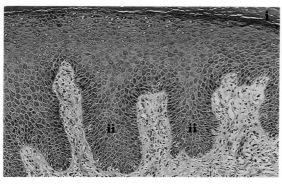

Fig. 4.2 Acanthosis

Acanthosis means thickening of the epidermis, mainly as a result of an increase in thickness of the prickle cell layer. There is usually an increase in the thickness of the basal and granular cell layers too and acanthosis is often associated with hyperkeratosis (i) (see Fig. 4.14). The acanthotic epidermis may be uniformly thickened, but there is usually disproportionate expansion of the rete ridges or 'pegs' (ii). Acanthosis is a commonly seen feature in many chronic inflammatory skin conditions, including chronic dermatitis (see Fig. 5.2), and psoriasis (see Fig. 6.2). 'Acanthoma' is the name applied to a localized thickening of the epidermis to produce a tumour-like mass. Examples of this usage are *clear cell acanthomas* (see Fig. 20.14) and pilar sheath acanthoma.

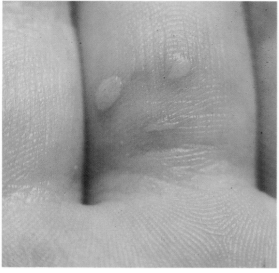

(a)

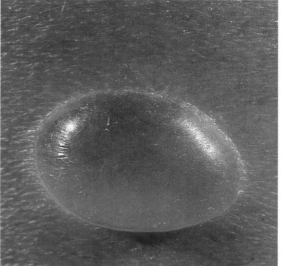

(b)

Fig. 4.3(a) & (b) Blisters: vesicles and bullae
These are fluid-filled lesions, a vesicle being less than 5 mm in diameter and a bulla greater than 5 mm, and they may be intra-epidermal or subepidermal. The appearance of a blister is largely related to the mechanical strength of adjacent skin: hence subepidermal blisters are tense in pemphigoid, when they require considerable pressure on them to spread laterally, but flaccid in toxic epidermal necrolysis when adjacent epidermis can easily be sheared by finger pressure (Nikolsky's sign). However, only subepidermal blisters will contain blood. The level at which the bulla has originated can be of value in histological diagnosis; this is tabulated and illustrated in Chapter 8.

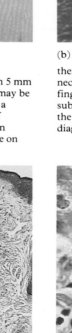

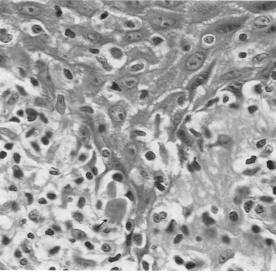

Fig. 4.4 Caseation
This is the name given to a histologically characteristic pattern of tissue necrosis in which the necrotic tissue is amorphous, homogeneous and pink-staining on H & E, with no ghost cell outlines or nuclear debris. To the naked eye, the necrotic material looks like white cream cheese, hence the name. This type of necrosis is largely confined to tuberculosis and gummatous lesions of tertiary syphilis; perversely, caseation is not a prominent feature of tuberculous skin lesions (lupus vulgaris: see Fig. 11.1(b), but in the skin is best seen in the non-tuberculous lesion, lupus miliaris disseminata faciei, as here.

Fig. 4.5 Colloid (or Civatte) Bodies
These small, spherical eosinophilic bodies are seen in the lower epidermis and upper dermis in a number of conditions in which there is hydropic degeneration of the basal cells of the epidermis (see Fig. 4.15), particularly when the damage is marked and long-standing. The two conditions in which they are seen most frequently are lichen planus and lupus erythematosus. They represent the remnants of dead basal cells.

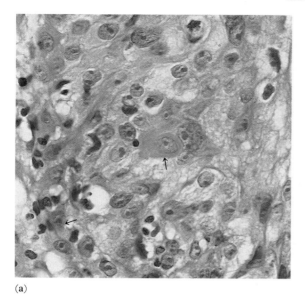

(a)

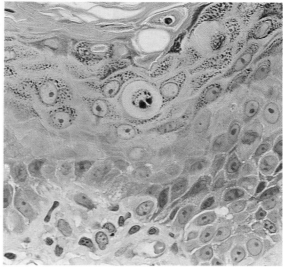

(b)

Fig. 4.6(a) & (b) Dyskeratosis

To the histopathologist this term describes abnormal patterns of keratinization in keratinocytes; it is a common feature of many neoplastic proliferations of squamous epithelial cells from many sites and is frequently seen in skin conditions such as the various types of intra-epidermal carcinoma and invasive squamous carcinoma. In addition, dyskeratosis may be seen as a result of disordered non-neoplastic proliferations of epidermis such as keratoacanthoma and some other pseudocarcinomatous epidermal hyperplasias. The term is also used by dermatologists to describe an assorted group of conditions in which there is disordered production of keratin (see Ch. 17). *Corps ronds* are the remains of degenerate

dyskeratotic epidermal cells which probably result from dyskeratosis within an epidermis in which an acantholytic process is occurring (see Fig. 4.1). Corps ronds are thus found in acantholytic disorders such as Darier's disease (see Fig. 17.5) and warty dyskeratoma (see Fig. 17.6). Micrograph (a) shows dyskeratosis of individual neoplastic keratinocytes within an intra-epidermal carcinoma (arrow). This probably represents premature keratinization of an immature neoplastic keratinocyte (individual cell keratinization). Micrograph (b) shows corps ronds from a case of Darier's disease. The central nucleus is pyknotic and is separated from the peripheral intracellular keratin by a variable pale-staining halo.

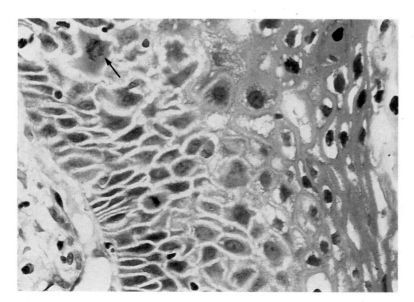

Fig. 4.7 Dysplasia

This term is applied to the cytological appearance of cells in which cytoplasmic and nuclear appearances are abnormal and indicative of disordered growth and maturity. The major abnormality in dysplastic cells is in the nucleus; there is variation in nuclear size and shape (nuclear pleormorphism) and increased intensity of nuclear staining (nuclear hyperchromicity) due to an increase in DNA content. There is an increase in mitoses, and abnormal mitotic figures such as tripolar mitoses (arrow) may be present. This micrograph shows dysplastic epidermal cells in solar keratosis; epithelial dysplasia is usually indicative of a neoplastic process, and is the main cytological characteristic of a malignant tissue.

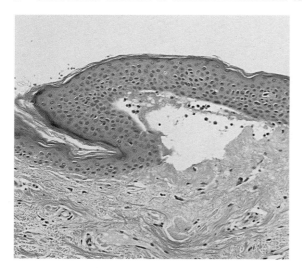

Fig. 4.8 Epidermolysis

This simply means separation of the epidermis, either from underlying epidermis (intra-epidermal split) or dermis (subepidermal split). The causes are numerous, and apparent clinically as a vesicle or bulla, as an erosion, or as a fold of sheared epidermis.

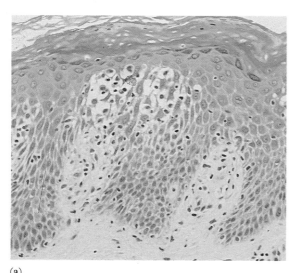

(a)

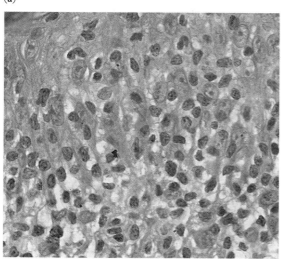

(b)

Fig. 4.9(a) & (b) Exocytosis and epidermotropism

Exocytosis is the term used to describe the invasion of the epidermis by chronic inflammatory cells (mainly lymphocytes) in association with spongiosis and vesiculation of epidermal cells. It is a common histological feature in inflammatory skin disease of many aetiologies; spongiotic vesiculation leads to oozing and parakeratotic scaling.

Epidermotropism is the descriptive term which has been used to describe the presence of lymphocytoid cells, singly or in small clumps, within the epidermis, but without associated spongiosis. It is not a feature of inflammatory skin disease, but is seen mainly in cutaneous T cell lymphoma, where the small clumps of lymphoid cells are known as Pautrier microabscesses. Micrograph (a) shows typical exocytosis in subacute dermatitis; note the associated spongiosis. Micrograph (b) shows epidermotropism of T lymphocytes into the epidermis in mycosis fungoides; note the absence of significant associated spongiosis (see also Figs. 22.2, 22.5(d)).

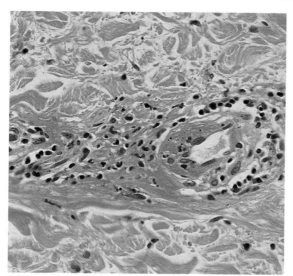

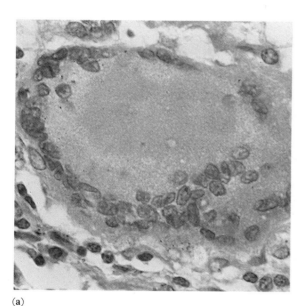

(a)

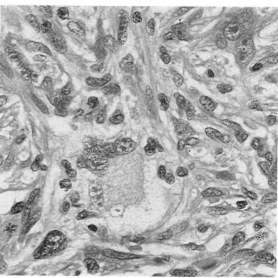

(b)

Fig. 4.10 Fibrinoid necrosis

'Fibrinoid' is an amorphous eosinophilic material composed of precipitated or polymerized plasma proteins, not all of which is polymerized fibrinogen (fibrin). It is seen most commonly in the walls of blood vessels which have undergone necrosis (fibrinoid necrosis), and in the skin is usually a histological finding in cases of acute vasculitis irrespective of the aetiology (e.g. drug-related, connective tissue disorder). This micrograph shows fibrinoid necrosis of an upper dermal blood vessel in a patient with acute vasculitis due to polyarteritis nodosa, (see also Fig. 12.2). The term fibrinoid degeneration is sometimes used to describe the alteration in staining characteristics of patches of upper dermal collagen seen in the acute lesion of systemic lupus erythematosus (see Fig. 9.); the collagen becomes amorphous and strongly eosinophilic. There is no evidence that fibrin or other plasma protein derivatives are present in SLE.

Fig. 4.11(a) & (b) Giant cells

The term giant cells is used to describe large cells with multiple nuclei; size alone does not entitle a cell to be described as giant. There are many types of multinucleate giant cells, the most common of which are derived from macrophages or histiocytes, but multinucleated giant epithelial and naevus cells also occur.

The so-called *Langhans-type giant cell*, seen in micrograph (a), has a large, central, homogenous, pale-pink-staining centre, and the nuclei are arranged in a ring around the periphery. Although classically described in association with tuberculosis, these cells are also found in sarcoidosis, foreign-body reactions, and in a number of other reactions. Multinucleate giant cells formed in response to the presence of a foreign body are less regular than those in TB or sarcoid, and the nuclei may be haphazardly scattered through the cell; the foreign body may also be visible in the cytoplasm of the giant cell. They are usually found as a component of a granulomatous type of chronic inflammatory reaction, a response to bacteria or other foreign material which cannot be destroyed or neutralised by neutrophil polymorphs.

The *Touton-type giant cell*, seen in micrograph (b), has a central, homogenous, dark-pink-staining centre surrounded by a ring of nuclei, outside of which is a peripheral rim of pale, foamy cytoplasm. They are only seen in various cutaneous xanthomatous lesions such as juvenile xanthogranuloma (see Fig. 23.4), since the Touton cell is nothing more than a multinucleate lipid-laden histiocyte (foam cell).

Epithelial multinucleate giant cells may be seen in the epidermis in herpes infections, and in some pleomorphic malignant epithelial tumours (see Fig. 18.4). *Multinucleate giant naevus cells* are seen in Spitz naevus (see Fig. 19.7). and in some malignant melanomas.

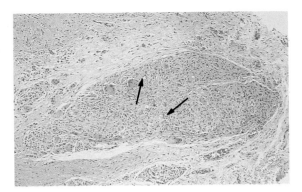

Fig. 4.12 Granuloma

A granuloma is a localized chronic inflammatory tissue response composed of histiocytes and lymphocytes, some of the histiocytes being large and multinucleated (giant cells). Such a reaction occurs in response to certain infections (e.g. TB), some fungi, and a wide range of foreign material, as well as sarcoid (see Fig. 11.3). Certain specific histological features may enable the cause of the granulomatous reaction to be identified, but often other means, e.g. microbiological culture, are necessary.

The photomicrograph shows a typical giant cell granuloma; in this case the cause is refractile inorganic material (arrows).

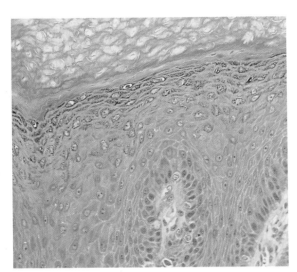

Fig. 4.13(a) & (b) Hypergranulosis and hypogranulosis

Hypergranulosis, seen in micrograph (a), describes an increase in thickness of the granular layer of the epidermis (stratum granulosum); this layer, which contains keratohyaline granules, is normally only one or two layers thick, but may become thicker in conditions of epidermal hyperplasia. Consequently, it is usually seen in association with acanthosis (see Fig. 4.1) and orthokeratotic hyperkeratosis; see Figure 4.14 (a). A thick granular layer is a normal feature of the thick skin at the extremities, e.g. soles.

Reduction or absence of the granular layer (hypogranulosis) seen in micrograph (b) is always abnormal and is associated with parakeratotic hyperkeratosis; see Figure. 4.14 (b). Further examples of hypergranulosis and hypogranulosis can be seen in many other illustrations in this book.

(a)

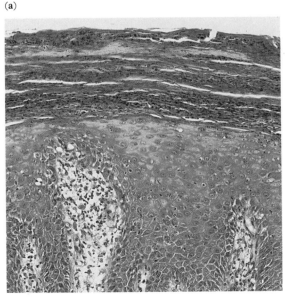

(b)

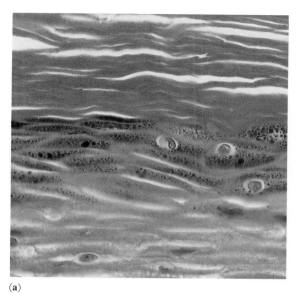

(a)

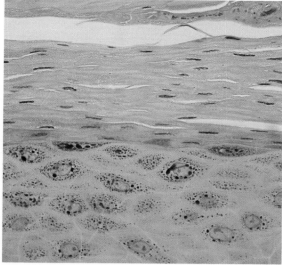

(b)

Fig. 4.14(a) & (b) Hyperkeratosis: orthokeratosis and parakeratosis

Hyperkeratosis is the thickening of the horny layer of keratin on the skin surface. If the thickened horny layer is composed of thin flakes of red-staining keratin which are devoid of any purple- or black-staining pyknotic nuclear debris, the term *orthokeratosis* is used. Micrograph 4.14(a) shows orthokeratotic hyperkeratosis.

When normal epidermal maturation is disturbed, as in some inflammatory skin conditions such as psoriasis, the granular layer is reduced in thickness or lost, and the overlying horny layer shows parakeratosis, seen in micrograph (b), in which the horny layer is composed of keratin flakes in which pyknotic nuclear remnants, usually flattened, are present.

Clinically hyperkeratosis appears as surface scaliness; the scales are particularly opaque and silver-white if there is parakeratosis.

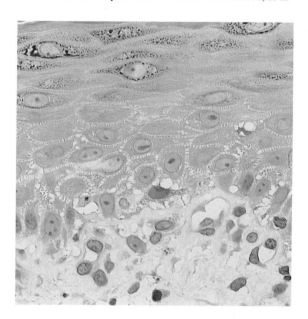

Fig. 4.15 Hydropic basal cell degeneration

This describes a pattern of epidermal abnormality which is confined to very few conditions, mainly lichen planus (see Fig. 7.2) and lupus erythematosus (see Figs. 9.1, 9.2). Histologically, there is swelling and vacuolation of basal cell cytoplasm due to intracellular accumulation of water (hence hydropic), followed by death of the basal cell. Continuing damage of this sort leads to loss of definition of the dermo-epidermal junction, often associated with a heavy chronic inflammatory cell infiltrate closely applied to the area of damage. Melanin from the damaged basal cell layer drops into the upper dermis (pigment incontinence) where it is phagocytosed by upper dermal macrophages (melanophages). Another consequence of basal layer damage is the presence of colloid or civatte bodies (see Fig. 4.5).

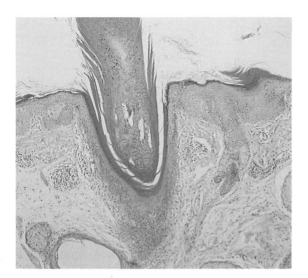

Fig. 4.16 Keratotic follicular plugging
Plugging of the dilated openings of hair follicles by masses of keratin is a feature of a limited number of skin conditions, particularly chronic discoid lupus erythematosus (see Fig. 9.2), Keratotic plugs may also block the mouths of sweat glands in ichthyosis vulgaris.

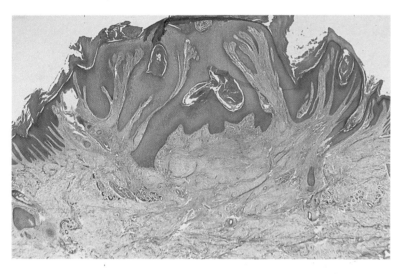

Fig. 4.17 Papillomatosis
This term is used to describe the histological appearance of exaggeration of the dermal papillae, throwing both the dermo-epidermal junction and the upper epidermal surface into exaggerated folds or undulations. It is a common feature of a number of chronic inflammatory skin disorders such as chronic psoriasis, but in these cases the distortion of the upper surface rarely reflects the degree of convolution of the dermo-epidermal juction. Papillomatosis is seen at its most florid in some viral warts (see Fig. 10.2), acanthosis nigricans (see Fig. 17.2) and epidermal naevi (see Fig. 20.3).

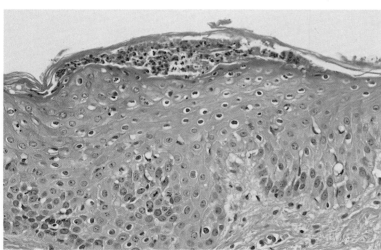

Fig. 4.18 Pustule
This is a localized collection of neutrophils beneath or within the epidermis; pustules are usually 1–3 mm in diameter although they may coalesce. Histologically, the lesion is a collection within the epidermis of neutrophils (or less commonly eosinophils) suspended in a variable amount of fluid. The location of the pustule within the epidermis may assist diagnosis; the illustrated example is a sub-corneal pustule.

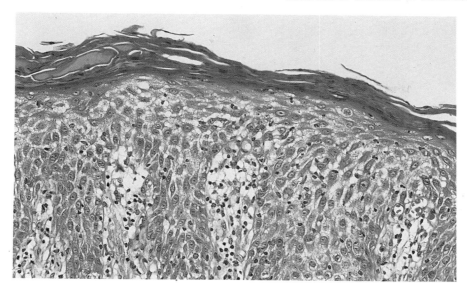

Fig. 4.19 Spongiosis

Focal intercellular oedema of the epidermis leads to separation of the epidermal cells, particularly in the prickle cell layer; this condition is known as spongiosis. Accumulation of fluid between epidermal cells causes gaps to appear which may coalesce to form fluid-filled vesicles (see Figs. 5.1, 8.1). Spongiosis is often associated with local exocytosis of inflammatory cells from the underlying dermis.

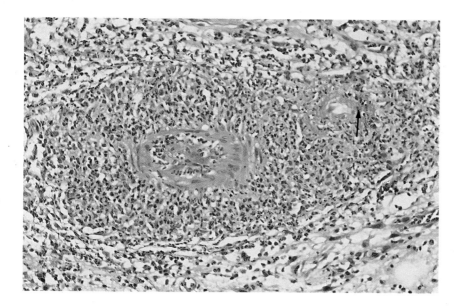

Fig. 4.20 Vasculitis

This term means inflammation of a vessel wall, and is the basis of many skin conditions, the more common of which are discussed and illustrated in Chapter 12. Vasculitis may be complicated by extravasation of blood, exudation of fibrin into and around the vessel wall (fibrinoid necrosis: see Fig. 4.10), and by thrombosis of the vessel lumen (see Fig. 12.2(d)). In this example a medium-sized artery from a case of polyarteritis nodosa shows destruction of the vessel wall by an inflammatory infiltrate, mainly neutrophils; there is focal fibrinoid necrosis (arrow).

5. Dermatitis

Introduction

The terms dermatitis and eczema are used synonymously. In simple terms, dermatitis implies inflammatory changes in the skin, namely vascular dilatation leading to clinical erythema, with exudation of plasma and inflammatory cells from the vessels into the surrounding dermis to produce swelling, clinically manifest as papules or oedematous plaques. In some cases the exudation of fluid and cells extends into the epidermis to produce spongiosis and vesicle formation. Conditions such as lichen planus, impetigo and psoriasis are also inflammatory diseases of skin, but are not generally understood when the term dermatitis is used, for they have either a recognizable and distinct histological pattern, e.g. psoriasis, or their pathogenesis is histologically obvious, e.g. impetigo. Lack of specific histological features has led to the use of the phrase 'non-specific dermatitis' to reflect the pathological anonymity of the inflammatory changes in many cases. As different exogenous and endogenous factors can produce the histological changes of non-specific dermatitis, the elucidation of the cause in any individual case is a task for the clinician rather than the histopathologist.

HISTOLOGICAL PATTERNS OF DERMATITIS

Histologically, three main patterns of non-specific dermatitis can be recognized:

1. Acute;
2. Sub-acute;
3. Chronic.

Fig.5.1(a) & (b) Acute dermatitis (*illustrations opposite*)
In acute dermatitis, the histological features of an acute inflammatory reaction, as seen elsewhere in the body, are seen at their best, and clinically the skin exhibits the cardinal signs of inflammation, calor (heat) rubor (erythema), tumour (swelling) and dolor (pain, often in the form of itch). Clinically, the appearance of the lesion is very mixed; there is usually a base of erythema or a raised indurated plaque which is not sharply delineated but merges gradually with surrounding skin. Vesicle formation is frequent in early stages, and may coalesce to form substantial blisters which frequently rupture with oozing of clear fluid and the formation of surface crust, as seen in (a). It is to this blistering, bubbling lesion, seen in the early stages of a severe eruption, that the term eczema (boiling out) was applied. Mild early lesions show only erythema and perhaps pin-point vesiculation, but these appearances, like those of the severe blistering pattern, are soon modified by secondary changes due to scratching, e.g. excoriations, urtication, fissuring etc. Persistence of the eruption, and continued trauma, leads to the features of a chronic dermatitis, i.e. lichenification, hyperkeratosis, and hardening of the skin (see Fig. 5.2).

As with all rashes, the clinical appearance varies with the site. For example, vesicle formation is easily seen on the palms and soles, but there is little oedema because the skin is tightly bound to underlying fascia; also the epidermis is thick at these sites and has an increased capacity for fluid.

Histologically, the basis of the erythema is a perivascular accumulation of inflammatory cells around dilated, often congested, upper dermal blood vessels, in which the endothelial cells may be swollen and almost cuboidal. Occasional neutrophils may be seen adherent to the swollen endothelial cells in some vessels, but around the vessel the predominant cell is the lymphocyte, with some macrophages and, in some acute dermatitic lesions with a contact allergic cause, a few eosinophils. The erythematous skin is usually raised above the level of adjacent normal skin because of oedema in the upper dermis, and this oedema is particularly obvious around the dilated blood vessels. In acute dermatitis, there is invariably migration of the inflammatory cells away from the perivascular regions up into papillary dermis and into the overlying epidermis (exocytosis). In areas where this migration of inflammatory cells into epidermis is most marked, there develops spongiosis which eventually becomes so marked as to produce vesicles which can coalesce to produce blisters. In acute irritant contact dermatitis, the epidermal cells may also show marked intracellular oedema; this, combined with the intercellular spongiotic oedema, may produce a pattern of blisters associated with reticular degeneration of the epidermis (see pp. 57, 61). In this circumstance, necrosis of epidermal cells is a frequently observed feature. Although the epidermis is expanded by fluid, vesicle formation and blistering, there is no acanthosis or hyperkeratosis, the skin surface often being partly coated with a proteinaceous crust derived from burst blisters; this pink-staining amorphous crust usually contains the pyknotic nuclear debris of dead inflammatory cells. If the lesions have been scratched, the crust may contain neutrophils or neutrophil nuclear debris. If secondary infection has supervened following scratching and rupturing of the blisters, neutrophils may be numerous and can be seen in the dermis beneath the excoriation.

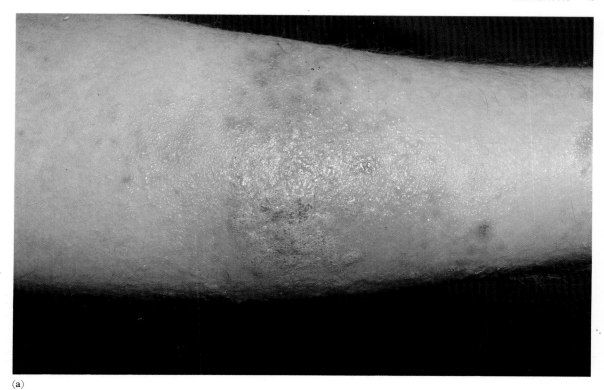

(a)

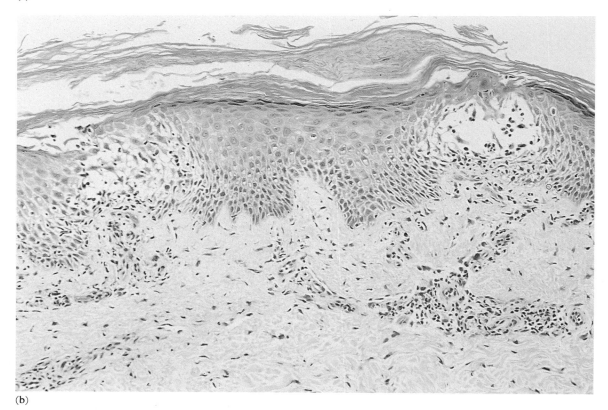

(b)

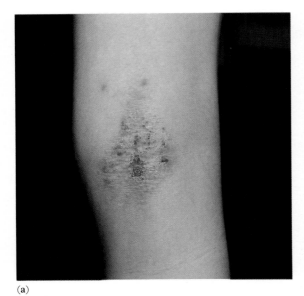

(a)

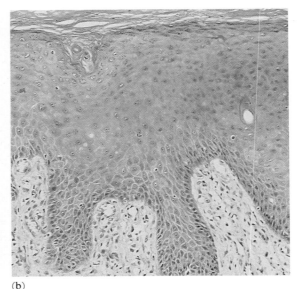

(b)

Fig. 5.2(a), (b) & (c) Chronic dermatitis

Clinically, in chronic dermatitis there is variable erythema, insignificant in old lesions, combined with lichenification and scaling, and increased pigmentation. Fissuring may be seen, as in (a). However, vesiculation and large blisters are absent.

Histologically, there is a perivascular lymphocytic infiltrate around upper dermal blood vessels which often appear rather thick-walled. There is variable spread of mixed chronic inflammatory cells into the dermis, including lymphocytes, plasma cells and macrophages, some of which contain melanin (melanophages). However, the upper dermis can show marked fibroblastic proliferation, particularly in the thickened papillae; vertical orientation of collagen fibres in the papillary dermis is an almost invariable finding. The epidermis is usually markedly thickened, with acanthosis, papillomatosis and overlying hyperkeratosis in which localized patches of parakeratosis are invariable. There is patchy hypergranulosis.

Micrograph (b) shows a largely inactive chronic dermatitis. Note the marked acanthosis, dermal fibrosis and prominent vessels. Micrograph (c) shows a chronic dermatitis in which some residual activity persists. Note the mild spongiosis, continuing exocytosis of inflammatory cells, dermal melanophages, and verticalization of dermal collagen.

Chronic dermatitis represents an end stage of long-standing, incompletely resolved acute or sub-acute dermatitis, modified by repeated trauma from rubbing or scratching. Because of its duration and lichenified appearance, this lesion has been called lichen simplex chronicus; any chronically rubbed skin lesion may produce histological appearances identical to those described above.

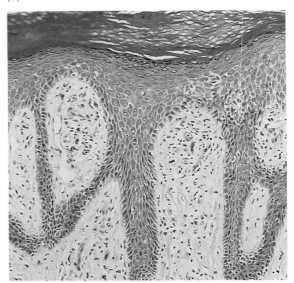

(c)

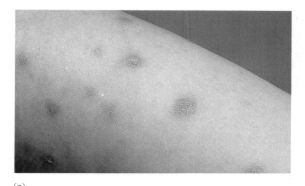

(a)

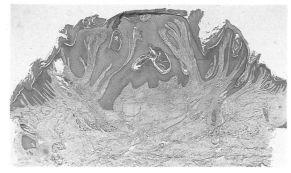

(b)

Fig. 5.3(a) & (b) Prurigo nodularis

This is a localized form of chronic dermatitis, usually produced by constant rubbing or picking of a single itchy papule. It consists of firm, often excoriated, dermal nodules with lichenification. Their distribution corresponds with intensity of scratching, so they are commonest on the limbs and front of chest and abdomen. The disease is usually unremitting. A frequently observed histological feature in prurigo nodularis lesions is hypertrophy, and often

proliferation, of dermal nerves. These lesions often remain intensely itchy and are consequently scratched frequently, leading to repeated episodes of surface ulceration ('picker's nodule'). Continuous cycles of ulceration and healing lead to very marked irregular epidermal acanthosis, such that the broad irregular rete ridges may have a pseudocarcinomatous appearance. Biopsied after recent trauma, a picker's nodule can show necrosis of upper epidermal layers, excoriation and crust formation.

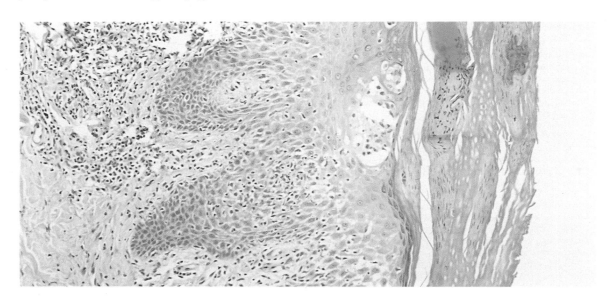

Fig. 5.4 Subacute dermatitis

This pattern shows some histological features of both acute and chronic dermatitis, and would probably be more accurately named 'chronic active' dermatitis, as is the practice with colitis and hepatitis at equivalent stages of their natural history.

Clinically, there is again raised erythema but blister formation is not marked. Small pin-point vesicles are visible in a moderately thickened epidermis. Discoid dermatitis (see Fig. 5.7) is a good example of subacute dermatitis.

Histologically, subacute dermatitis again shows a perivascular accumulation of lymphocytes and histiocytes in the upper dermis, but the vessels are less dilated than in acute dermatitis, and there is less perivascular and dermal oedema and vessel endothelial swelling. The chronic inflammatory cell infiltrate is more localized to the

perivascular region, and spread of inflammatory cells into upper dermis and epidermis is less marked. The epidermis shows moderate thickening due to acanthosis, with some elongation of rete ridges; spongiosis is focal, any spongiotic vesicles being small with little tendency to fuse together to form large blisters. Exocytosis of inflammatory cells is largely confined to the areas of spongiosis and microvesiculation. There is rarely significant hyperkeratosis, but small mounds of parakeratosis may occur in the keratin layer over the spongiotic vesicles. Thus, histologically, subacute dermatitis shows features of both acute dermatitis (e.g. spongiosis, vesiculation and exocytosis) and chronic dermatitis (e.g. acanthosis and papillomatosis). This is the pattern in discoid dermatitis; the plaques are raised partly as a result of dermal oedema and partly because of epidermal thickening.

CLINICAL PATTERNS OF DERMATITIS

Dermatitis can result from many causes, which may interact. The commonest types are atopic dermatitis, contact irritant and contact allergic dermatitis, discoid dermatitis and gravitational dermatitis. Seborrhoeic dermatitis is now widely thought to be a direct result of infection with *Pityrosporum* but is discussed here.

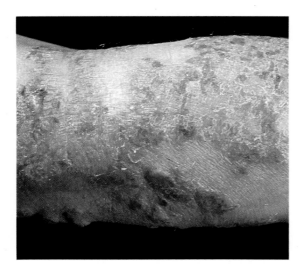

Fig. 5.5 Atopic dermatitis

This usually first presents in infancy with symmetrical eruptions on the face, but later involves the trunk and limbs, particularly the antecubital fossae, popliteal fossae and other flexures. Clinically, there is raised erythema, with weeping and scaling, but the appearances are modified by the effects of scratching since the lesions are itchy from the outset. Hence the clinical and pathological features of chronic dermatitis quickly supervene on the original acute dermatitic changes. The presence of pustules and crusting indicates secondary infection by bacteria, usually staphylococci or streptococci introduced during scratching. There is often a family history of atopic dermatitis or asthma in a parent or sibling; failing that , one of the parents may be prone to hay-fever or urticaria.

Fig. 5.6(a) & (b) Contact dermatitis

There are two main types of contact dermatitis: *primary irritant dermatitis* where the skin is damaged as a direct toxic effect of the agent, and *allergic contact dermatitis* in which skin damage is produced by immunological mechanisms, the contact agent acting as an hapten.

Primary irritant dermatitis can occur in anyone in contact with strong agents, particularly alkalis and detergents, hence housewives, hairdressers and industrial workers are particularly prone. Allergic contact dermatitis occurs in people with a predisposition, possibly inherited; common agents producing the reaction include nickel, rubber, cosmetics and some dyes. In some cases an allergic dermatitis is triggered by the combination of exposure to an allergen and exposure to light (photoallergic dermatitis).

Figure 5.6(a) shows a primary irritant dermatitis to shampoo in a young hairdresser while (b) shows an allergic contact dermatitis to a nickel stud on a belt.

In this group of disorders, erythema, oedema and blistering are often extreme, and the histological appearances are those of an acute dermatitis (see Fig. 5.1), initially localized to the area of contact but often spreading subsequently. Previous contact results in the same changes already described in chronic atopic dermatitis, i.e. erythema and lichenification.

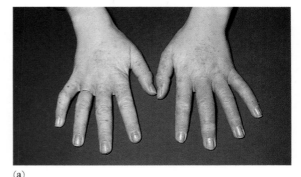

(a)

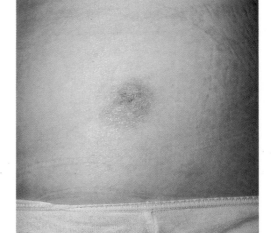

(b)

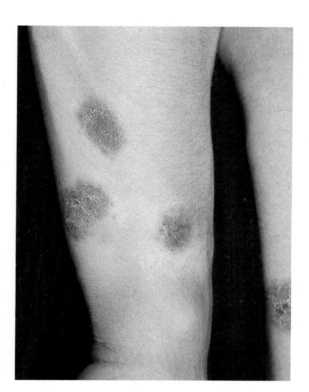

Fig. 5.7 Discoid dermatitis

This is most common in middle-aged and elderly men and presents as several rounded, 2–5 cm coin-shaped areas of raised red skin bearing tiny vesicles and papules. The edges of the lesion are characteristically sharply defined, and scaling, if present, is evenly spread across the surface. In elderly men, these lesions occur mainly on the trunk and extensor surfaces of the limb; less commonly, it may occur in young women when it is mainly seen on the dorsal surfaces of hands and fingers. The lesions are intensely itchy, so the tiny vesicles are often traumatized and deroofed, allowing their fluid to ooze onto the skin surface to produce crusting; scratching predisposes to secondary bacterial infection, and the lesions are often crusted and secondarily infected with *Staphylococci* at first presentation.

Although lesions can become chronic, recurrent crops of acute lesions is the usual pattern.

Discoid dermatitis histologically shows the features of a subacute or chronic active dermatitis (see Fig. 5.4) with small spongiotic vesicles in the epidermis as an indicator of continuing activity. However, the persistence of the lesions, and the result of constant scratching, leads to the development of the histological features of a chronic dermatitis. The cause is unknown.

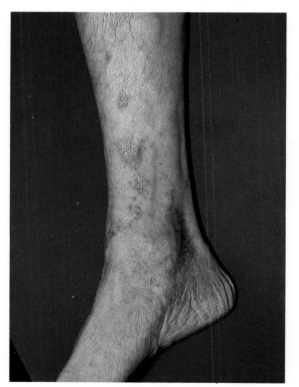

Fig. 5.8 Gravitational dermatitis

Early signs are lower leg oedema, induration and brown-grey pigmentation; this may progress to ulceration and atrophy with a solid feel due to extensive subcutaneous and dermal fibrosis. It is most common in patients with varicose veins.

The histological appearances in gravitational dermatitis are complex because of the associated dermal changes of chronic venous insufficiency, viz. proliferation of thick-walled vessels, dense dermal fibrosis, red cell extravasation and haemosiderin deposition. The clinically observed skin induration, atrophy and brown pigmentation are the result of chronic venous insufficiency rather than dermatitis. The dermatitic features are erythema, oedema and scaling; these changes are seen at their most severe when there is superimposed contact dermatitis due to topical treatment, when there may be severe vesiculation and blistering.

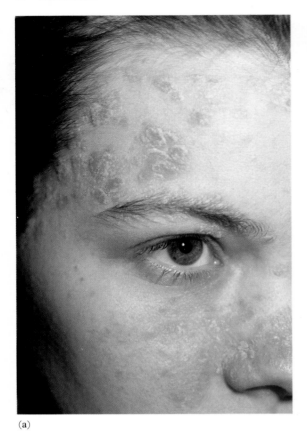

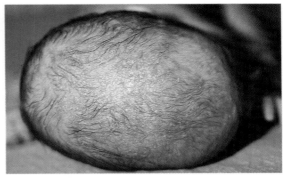

(b)

(a)

Fig. 5.9(a) & (b) Seborrhoeic dermatitis

This usually presents with erythema and characteristic greasy scaling on the central face, eyebrows, scalp, around the ears, central chest and back.

In infants, the first manifestation of the disease is the presence on the scalp of waxy yellowish scales, often thick and confluent, and difficult to remove from the scalp and hair ('cradle cap'), as seen in (b). The skin inflammation spreads down onto the face, particularly around the eyebrows and ears. An identical rash may originate in the napkin area but extends up on to the trunk and into the axillae.

In adult-pattern seborrhoeic dermatitis the scalp and face are again commonly involved. The scalp shows excessive white scaling associated with variable skin erythema; the face, the cheeks, side of the nose and forehead are the common sites, as seen in (a). Less commonly the rash occurs on the trunk and intertrigenous regions, the latter particularly in obese people.

The erythema is the result of dilatation of upper dermal capillaries which are cuffed by lymphocytes and histiocytes, with a few neutrophils. The scale is composed of excess ortho- and parakeratotic keratin containing clumps of neutrophils, the latter being most obvious in the horny layer around plugged follicles. There is usually some acanthosis and mild spongiosis. In chronic seborrhoeic dermatitis the acanthosis often has a psoriasiform pattern.

The disease is probably caused by skin infection with *Pityrosporum* yeasts.

Fig. 5.10 Artefactual dermatitis

Self-inflicted dermatitis can be difficult to diagnose clinically, particularly when the patient is plausible, as is often the case. Lesions are most frequent on the face, hands and arms, and usually consist of recent and old excoriations, often linear or in a bizarre pattern. In long-standing trauma, nodular prurigo lesions and scars may be present. All of these features are seen in this example. Histologically, the picture is confusing; the presence of a number of epidermal excoriations of varying ages, associated with a disproportionately scanty dermal inflammatory infiltrate, is usually the only histological clue to the diagnosis. However, it is important to exclude a valid reason for scratching, such as increased numbers of dermal eosinophils.

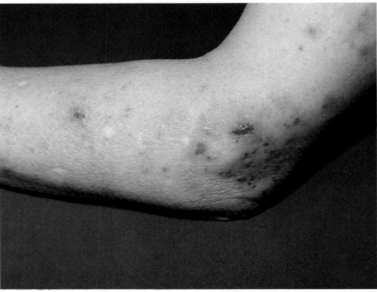

(c)

Pathogenesis of dermatitis

Histological examination only occasionally gives any indication of the pathogenesis of a non-specific dermatitis in the acute and subacute stages, and almost never in the chronic stage. Fine subtleties of histological variation are usually of no pathogenetic significance, often being more a manifestation of secondary traumatic effects.

Occasionally, the nature of the cellular content of the infiltrate, or the severity of epidermal necrosis may offer clues. The presence of numerous eosinophils should raise the possibility of an allergic reaction to drugs, chemicals, fungi or fleas. If eosinophils are present in the epidermal infiltrate, other possibilities include dermatophyte infections, scabies, and possibly pemphigoid at a pre-bullous stage. The presence of numerous plasma cells should raise suspicions of syphilis. When epidermal cell necrosis is frequent, particularly near the surface, contact with an irritant or allergen is likely; primula dermatitis can show dramatic epidermal necrosis. Some drug-induced skin reactions, particularly of the erythema multiforme type, show epidermal cell necrosis, as do some phototoxic eruptions.

If no specific features are visible, it is always worth staining the sections by the PAS method or the Grocott-Gomori methenamine silver to look for fungal hyphae in the surface keratin (see Fig. 10.19) since the common dermatophytic fungi are difficult to see in a routine H & E-stained paraffin section. Finally, detailed examination of a skin biopsy at a number of levels greatly increases the chances of an accurate descriptive report, and may help point to an aetiology; for example, in some dermatitis lesions, spongiotic foci or vesicles may be few and far between and numerous levels may need to be examined before they are detected. Small patches of proteinaceous crust or foci of parakeratosis over an apparently normal epidermis should always stimulate the pathologist to examine deeper levels, as should unusual concentrations of inflammatory cells near the tip of a single papilla.

In the end, the pathologist has to report many such lesions as 'non-specific chronic (or acute, or subacute) dermatitis with no clue to its nature', and the onus is on the clinician to determine the cause or to classify it further.

6. Psoriasis and psoriasiform eruptions

Introduction

Psoriasis is a common relapsing and remitting condition which is characterized by well-circumscibed, red-pink or brown plaques covered by layers of silvery white scale which, when removed, reveal a large number of punctate vessels, some of which may bleed. Plaques are prominent on knees, elbows, trunk and scalp, and lose their scaly appearance in the flexures where they are smooth and glazed. Involvement of nail matrix results in nail dystrophy characterized by pitting and onycholysis. Inheritance appears to be polygenic. There are a number of other clinical variants (see Figs. 6.1 and 6.3).

A number of inflammatory skin conditions have some of the clinical and histological features of psoriasis; these are often imprecisely referred to as 'psoriasiform dermatitis'. Conditions such as some forms of seborrhoeic dermatitis, pityriasis rubra pilaris and some drug reactions (see Fig. 6.4) can mimic psoriasis clinically and histologically.

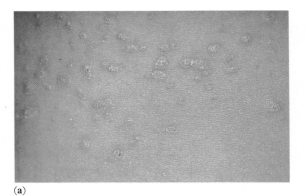

(a)

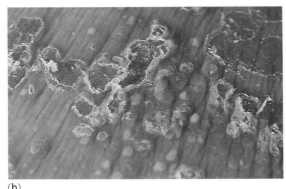

(b)

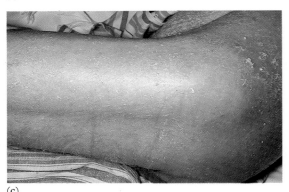

(c)

Fig. 6.1(a), (b) & (c). Important clinical variants of psoriasis

Figure 6.1(a) illustrates *guttate psoriasis* which appears as 0.5–1 cm, eruptive scaly plaques, usually in a child, sometimes following tonsillitis. (b) illustrates *erythrodermic psoriasis*, a dramatic illness with universal bright red erythema, sometimes with oedema. (c) illustrates *pustular psoriasis* which may be generalized as in the lesions shown here, or may be localized. A common pattern of localized pustular psoriasis is illustrated and discussed in Figure 6.3.

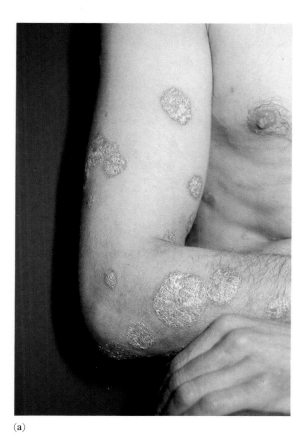

(a)

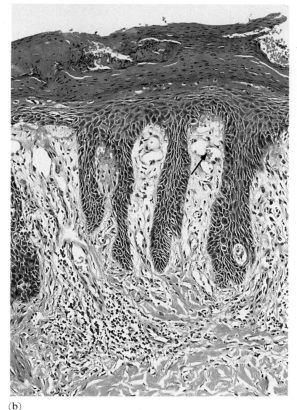

(b)

Fig. 6.2(a), (b) & (c). Classical psoriasis

Figure 6.2(a) shows typical lesions of classical psoriasis
located around the elbow. Note the sharply dermarcated red
plaque and the thick white scale. (b) shows the typical
histological appearances of an active psoriatic lesion,
equivalent to the expanding edge of a lesion shown in (a)
above. There is marked adherent parakeratosis within
which are occasional aggregates of pyknotic neutrophil
nuclei forming the Munro microabscesses characteristic of
active psoriasis. In general, the epidermis is thick as a result
of the elongation and broadening of the rete ridges;
however, between these enlarged rete ridges, the dermal
papillae are swollen by oedema and contain prominent
dilated capillaries (arrow). The epidermis over these club-
like papillae is extremely thin (suprapapillary thinning). In
these regions, the lifting off of the white scale
(parakeratosis) reveals the dilated capillaries at the tips of
the clubbed papillae in the form of minute red dots seen
through the translucent epidermis in the area of
suprapapillary thinning; clumsy removal of the scale also
tears away the thin epidermis leading to trauma of the
delicate swollen papillary dermis, producing punctate
bleeding from the dilated capillaries.

When Munro microabscesses are present in the
parakeratotic layer, as in (c), there is almost invariably a
scattering of neutrophils throughout the thin suprapapillary
epidermis; often the neutrophils aggregate in small clumps
to produce the so-called spongiform pustule of Kogoj. In
active psoriasis the epidermal cells show histological
evidence of rapid turnover, with mitotic activity above the
basal layer. There is usually no definable stratum

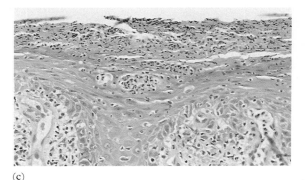

(c)

granulosum as keratohyaline granules are absent beneath
the area of parakeratosis. The upper dermis shows a mild
chronic inflammatory cell infiltrate.

It is the focal infiltration of the epidermis and overlying
parakeratotic keratin by neutrophils (spongiform pustule of
Kogoj and Munro microabscess respectively) which are the
characteristic histological features of psoriasis; rete ridge
enlargement, dermal papillary oedema and suprapapillary
epidermal thinning are seen in a number of other non-
psoriatic dermatoses, and are not specific.

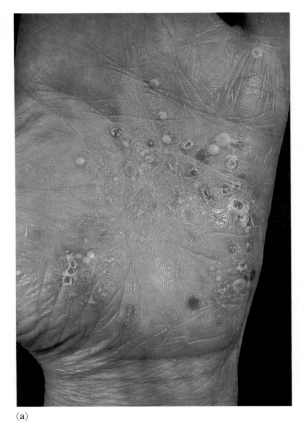

(a)

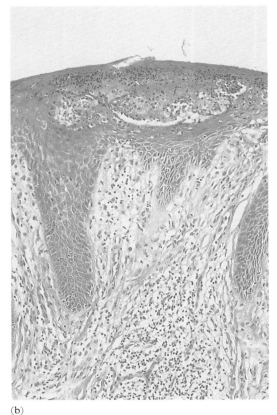

(b)

Fig. 6.3(a) & (b). Pustular psoriasis

Despite the prominence of neutrophils in and above the epidermis in psoriasis, and the frequency of small neutrophil aggregates, pustules are not usually visible to the naked eye. However, they are the predominant physical sign in pustular psoriasis of the palms and soles, characterized by successive crops of 2–3 mm epidermal pustules which are associated with prominent erythema, scaling and fissuring. In *generalized pustular psoriasis*, superficial pustules may arise in patients who have pre-existing psoriasis vulgaris, but may occur de novo as a severe generalized eruption of sudden onset. In *acrodermatitis continua*, pustules develop around nails, with erosions and peripheral scale. The nails may be destroyed; *pustulosis palmaris et plantaris* affects the palms of the hands and the soles of the feet, although rarely

other sites.

Figure 6.3(a) shows the typical clinical appearance of the pustules from a patient with pustular psoriasis of palms and soles.

Figure 6.3(b) shows an early lesion of pustular psoriasis in which there is a significant accumulation of neutrophils and fluid (forming a pustule) in the epidermis. The lesion is very focal, and adjacent epidermis is usually normal except for the occasional presence of small neutrophil nuclear aggregates at the edges of the large pustule; there is a scanty inflammatory cell infiltrate confined to the dermis underlying the pustule. This appearance is typical of the localized pustular psoriasis types; in the generalized types, the pustules are superimposed upon general psoriatic change.

Conditions which clinically and histologically resemble psoriasis

A number of dermatoses may show some of the histological features seen in psoriasis, particularly rete ridge elongation and clubbing, dermal papillary oedema with capillary dilatation and patchy exocytosis; seborrhoeic dermatitis, chronic erythroderma and exfoliative dermatitis, and some drug eruptions, are the commonest, and can usually be distinguished clinically. However, if spongiform pustules and Munro microabscesses are absent, and parakeratosis is not prominent, then psoriasis is unlikely. Another useful clue is that in psoriasis, the upper dermal chronic inflammatory cell infiltrate is disproportionately mild for the degree of epidermal abnormality. Eosinophils are rarely seen as a component of the upper dermal (and epidermal) infiltrate in psoriasis but may be numerous in some of the psoriasiform lesions, particularly the erythrodermatous lesions due to drugs. An example of a dermatosis which may resemble one of the clinical patterns of psoriasis is demonstrated in Figure 6.4.

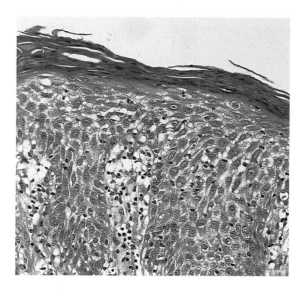

Fig. 6.4. Psoriasiform dermatitis (non-pustular)
This example, from a patient with a chronic erythrodermatous eruption, shows the following psoriasis-like features: acanthosis with elongation and clubbing of rete ridges, papillary oedema and capillary dilatation, some suprapapillary thinning, and parakeratotic scale. In addition, there are inflammatory cells in the epidermis, although spongiform pustules and Munro microabscesses are not present. This pattern may be difficult to distinguish from the erythrodermatous type of psoriasis, as may the early lesions of pityriasis rubra pilaris.

Pustular conditions such as impetigo (see Fig. 10.9), subcorneal pustular dermatosis and crusting lesions of Reiter's syndrome may be histologically almost impossible to distinguish from psoriasis, especially penile and nail lesions. Skin lesions of Reiter's syndrome (see Fig. 6.5) have many of the clinical features of psoriasis; the other disorders are clinically distinct.

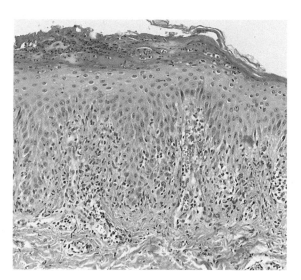

Fig. 6.5. Pustular psoriasiform lesion in Reiter's syndrome
This lesion was present on the glans penis (balanitis circinata) and shows many of the histological features of psoriasis. There is irregular acanthosis, papillary dermal oedema and hyperaemia, and neutrophil aggregates in the overlying parakeratosis.

7. Lichen planus, lichen nitidus and lichenoid eruptions

Introduction

Lichen planus is a self-limiting inflammatory condition of unknown aetiology, usually lasting between 6–17 months. It produces a quickly spreading eruption of itchy papules with characteristic morphology; they are sharply outlined, 2–5 mm across, polygonal, violet-pink, flat-topped and shiny. A diagnostic feature is the presence of Wickham's striae, which are fine white lines on the surface of the papule. The rash particularly affects the flexor aspects of the forearm, the wrists and ankles, and the lumbar region. It usually involves the oral mucosa (*buccal lichen planus*, see Fig. 7.6), and often the genitalia, On mucosal surfaces the clinical and histological appearances differ from those seen in skin lesions because mucosa is non-keratinizing; there is erythema and a superimposed lacy network of fine white lines and papules. Less common clinical variants of lichen planus include:

1. *Hypertrophic lichen planus* (see Fig. 7.3). This occurs most frequently on the shin; it is characterized by very persistent thick warty plaques of hyperkeratosis, usually with violaceous colour typical of lichen planus. It may be difficult to distinguish from lichen simplex chronicus.

2. *Follicular lichen planus* (*lichen planopilaris*) (see Fig. 7.4). This usually involves the scalp, and involvement of hair follicles in the disease leads to hair loss.

3. *Bullous lichen planus* (see Fig. 7.5). This is rare. It results from separation at the level of the damaged basal layer, resulting in bulla formation. It is most common on the legs and feet.

In addition to the above, three further changes are worthy of note: (i) erosion in lichen planus is fairly common in mucosal lesions, but is rare elsewhere; (ii) healing lichen planus often appears hyperpigmented (due to pigment incontinence resulting from long-standing damage to the basal layer). However, scarring is rare unless there has been ulceration; (iii) involvement of the nailfold in lichen planus may lead to longitudinal grooving, pterygium and nail atrophy or destruction.

The condition known as lichen nitidus (see Fig. 7.7) has some of the clinical and histological features seen in lichen planus, but it is not clear whether it is a variant of lichen planus, or a separate entity.

Lichenoid drug eruptions (see Fig. 7.8) are clinically and histologically so similar to lichen planus that they are better described as 'drug-induced lichen planus'.

A common histological thread through all the above lesions in their active phase is hydropic or liquefactive degeneration of the basal layer of epidermal cells. This distinctive histological change is also found in lupus erythematosus (see Figs. 9.1 and 9.2), and is an important diagnostic feature. It is also discussed and illustrated in Figure 4.15.

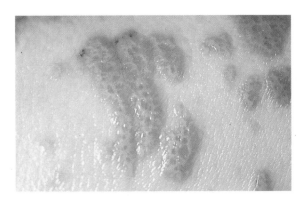

Fig. 7.1. Lichen planus
The photograph shows the classical appearance of lichen planus. The individual lesions start as small papules 1 to 2 mm across, which may enlarge and coalesce. In the early stages they are polygonal (because of the tendency of the lesions to be limited by skin creases) and shiny. The papules have a characteristic violaceous colour, often broken by a reticular pattern of white lines known as Wickham's striae; there is no satisfactory histological explanation for these characteristic striae.

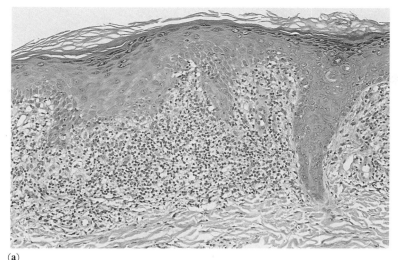

(a)

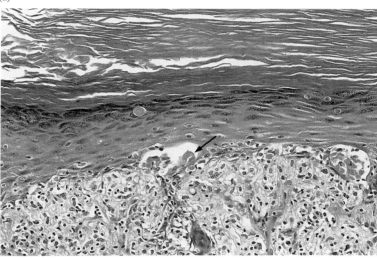

(b)

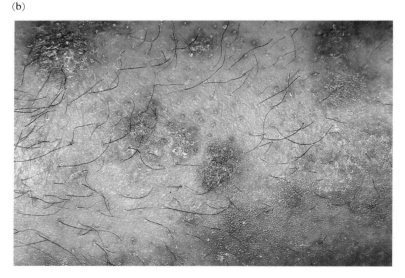

Fig. 7.2(a) & (b). Classical lichen planus

These micrographs show the typical histological features of classical lichen planus at a florid active stage. The five major features are:

1. Hyperkeratosis, parakeratosis being rare or absent;
2. Irregular thickening of granular layer;
3. Acanthosis, with irregular lengthening of rete ridges;
4. Dermal chronic inflammatory cell infiltrate, usually heavy and closely applied to dermo-epidermal border, with variable oedema;
5. Liquefaction or hydropic degeneration of epidermal basal layer.

In micrograph (b) advanced degeneration of the basal layer has produced a 'moth-eaten', indistinct dermo-epidermal junction containing round eosinophilic remnants of dead basal cells (colloid or Civatte bodies) (arrow).

The combination of irregular lengthening of rete ridges, basal layer destruction, and upper dermal oedema and inflammatory infiltrate, often produces a 'saw-tooth' appearance of rete ridges as seen in micrograph (a).

With the passage of time, the active destruction of the basal layers ceases. Colloid bodies become reduced in number or disappear although a few may remain in uppermost dermis, often in clumps of two or three. The basal layer may become reconstituted but remains irregular, with haphazardly arranged cells of varying sizes, for a long time. As the basal cell damage ceases, the chronic inflammatory infiltrate in the upper dermis becomes reduced both in intensity and in the crisp, band-like localization, acquiring a largely perivascular distribution; lymphocytes become less predominant and increased numbers of histiocytes appear. The changes in the epidermis vary; usually the epidermis becomes thinned (atrophic lichen planus) revealing the melanin within dermal macrophages beneath; the lesion may therefore show striking hyperpigmentation.

Fig. 7.3. Hypertrophic lichen planus

This occurs in the form of thick, warty plaques which usually occur on the shins. Although the typical changes of lichen planus are evident in the basal layer and upper dermis, there is epidermal thickening with acanthosis, papillomatosis and marked hyperkeratosis.

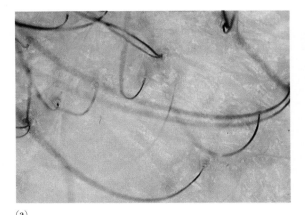

(a)

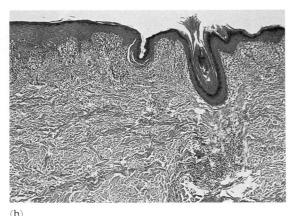

(b)

Fig. 7.4(a) & (b). Follicular lichen planus (lichen planopilaris)

This is most common on the scalp and neck where it produces red, scaly, pointed keratotic follicular papules, and eventually results in destruction of the hair follicles and hair loss, with scarring.

In addition to the histological features of classical lichen planus described and illustrated in Figure 7.2, in

lichen planopilaris, the chronic inflammatory cell infiltrate extends deeper into dermis around the hair follicles, the basal layer of which may also show hydropic degeneration. Affected follicles are dilated and contain a keratotic plug. Continuing inflammation leads to destruction of the hair follicle and hair, and in the latest stages the pilosebaceous apparatus disappears, leaving only dermal fibrosis and patchy dermal chronic inflammatory cell infiltrate.

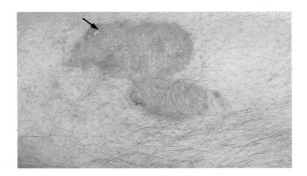

Fig. 7.5. Bullous lichen planus

In some lichen planus lesions, particularly those on the legs, excessive fluid accumulates at the site of the degenerating basal layer to form small subepidermal vesicles which frequently coalesce to form a bulla (arrow); it is uncommon. Rupture of the bulla produces ulceration and may lead to scarring. Histologically, this type of bulla is usually easy to distinguish from other causes, since the characteristic histological features of lichen planus are easily seen at the edges of the bulla.

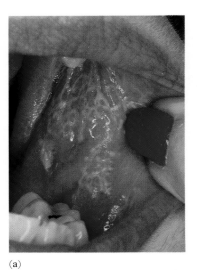

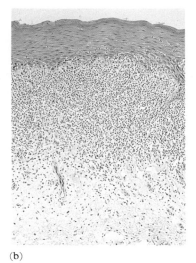

(a)   (b)

Fig. 7.6(a) & (b). Buccal lichen planus

Involvement of the oral mucosa in lichen planus produces reddish plaques showing a network of fine lacy white lines, erosions, and sometimes ulceration. Occasionally buccal lesions occur alone, without any associated skin involvement.

Lichen planus involving the buccal mucosa shows many of the classical features of lichen planus shown in Figure 7.2, including the important hydropic basal degeneration. There are, however, a number of differences, based upon the different structure and properties of oral squamous epithelium and skin epidermis. There is *no* focal thickening of the granular layer, which is not normally present in buccal mucosa, and parakeratosis is frequent. Atrophy of the epithelium is more common than in the skin.

(a)

Fig. 7.7(a) & (b). Lichen nitidus

The characteristic lesions are uniform, 1–2 mm in diameter, pink, flat-topped, sharply demarcated papules, usually on the penis, wrist and trunk; there are no Wickham's striae. Mucous membrane involvement is uncommon and, unlike lichen planus, the rash does not itch. It is much less common than classical lichen planus and the lesions persist for much longer.

This condition shows some of the important histological features of lichen planus, viz hydropic basal cell degeneration and upper dermal inflammatory cell infiltrate, but has a number of important histological differences:

1. Affected epidermis is thinned;
2. Inflammatory cells form an ill-defined nodule rather than a band, partly enclosed by rete ridges;
3. Inflammatory cells spill into overlying epidermis;
4. Overlying parakeratosis is almost invariable;
5. Histiocytes and giant cells may occur in infiltrate;
6. Colloid bodies are not seen in lichen nitidus.

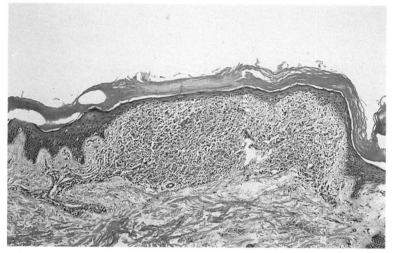

(b)

Fig. 7.8. Drug-induced lichen planus

Frequent causes include thiazide diuretics, gold and occasionally antimalarials; it may be provoked by sunlight. Histologically, the rash shows the features seen in classical lichen planus (see Fig. 7.2) from which it cannot be distinguished (see p. 112).

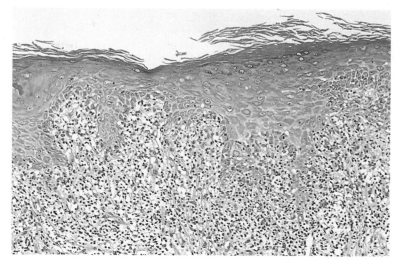

8.   Blistering and pustular disorders

Introduction

Many skin disorders which particularly affect the epidermis may produce fluid-filled blisters, either small (less than 5 mm diameter, termed vesicles) or larger (greater than 5 mm diameter termed bullae; see p. 32). Although the blister content is usually proteinaceous fluid, cells may be present, including degenerate or necrotic epidermal cells and inflammatory cells, usually neutrophils and eosinophils in variable proportions. When the blister content is comparatively cell-free, the fluid is usually clear, but increasing numbers of polymorphs make the fluid progressively cloudy until, with very large numbers of white cells, it becomes thick, opaque and creamy. Such a lesion is called a pustule; unlike most other examples of polymorph-rich fluid (pus) accumulation elsewhere in the body, pustule formation in the skin is *not* always a consequence of bacterial infection. Fluid accumulations within or at the base of the epidermis are usually the result of damage to the epidermal cells themselves, or to disruption of their attachments to each other and the epidermal basal lamina. In most cases the mechanism of epidermal or basal damage is not known, but infective (e.g. viral) and immunological causes are recognized, as are a number of inherited diseases in which skin blistering is a predominant feature. It is important to distinguish between those blisters which have originated within the epidermis above the basal layer (intra-epidermal) and those which have originated in the region of the basal cell layer and basal lamina at the dermo-epidermal junction (basal or subepidermal blister).

Intra-epidermal blisters can be further subdivided using two different criteria: (i) the level at which separation has occurred within the epidermis, and (ii) the nature of the process leading to the separation of epidermal cells.

Basal blisters can be approximately subdivided according to the type of inflammatory cell present in the blister fluid (see Table 8.2).

Accurate classification of a blister provides clues to the most likely diagnosis. This histological classification of the blistering process is summarized in Tables 8.1 and 8.2, and discussed in the following text.

INTRA-EPIDERMAL BLISTERS

Pathogenesis of intra-epidermal blisters

The sequence of histological changes which lead to intra-epidermal blister formation can usually be identified provided an early lesion is biopsied; at a later stage it may be impossible to determine the mechanism histologically.

Most intra-epidermal blisters arise as a consequence of three main processes, and this forms the basis of a useful histological classification. The three basic pathological processes are:

Spongiosis (see Fig. 4.19)

Mild spongiosis (fluid accumulation between epidermal cells) is a common feature of many inflammatory skin conditions, but when severe the fluid accumulation is such that a small intra-epidermal blister is formed (spongiotic vesicle). The mechanism rarely produces large bullae except by the fusion of adjacent vesicles to produce a confluent bulla. Spongiosis is usually associated with the migration (exocytosis; see p. 34) of inflammatory cells into the epidermis from the upper dermis, so spongiotic blisters often contain a mixture of small numbers of lymphocytes, neutrophils and occasionally eosinophils. As a general rule, spongiotic blisters with a high content of lymphocytes and/or eosinophils should lead one to suspect an allergic or immunological cause, whereas a predominant neutrophil component should raise the possibility of an infective cause. It is useful to subdivide spongiotic blisters into two categories, those with and those without pustule formation.

Acantholysis (see Fig. 4.1)

This process is the separation of adjacent epidermal cells due to disruption or dissolution of their attachments to each other and frequently leads to the formation of fluid-filled clefts, and later, vesicles and bullae. It is important to try to distinguish between primary and secondary acantholysis. In *primary acantholysis*, the epidermal cells appear normal at the onset of the acantholytic process and the extent of the separation is uniform throughout the early lesion. However, in the later stages of primary acantholysis, when a substantial bulla has formed, the separated acantholytic cells become histologically abnormal as a result of loss of attachments and of their altered fluid milieu, becoming rounded with dense spherical nuclei and intensely eosinophilic cytoplasm (acantholytic cells). Examples of lesions showing primary acantholysis are pemphigus vulgaris (see Fig. 8.3), benign familial pemphigus (see Fig. 8.4), Darier's disease (see Fig. 17.5), and warty dyskeratoma (see Fig. 17.6). In *secondary acantholysis*, the epidermal cells are histologically abnormal *before* significant separation occurs, and the separation appears to be a secondary phenomenon to epidermal cell damage. It may be seen in viral skin lesions (see Figs. 10.1(d), (e)) secondary to viral-induced epidermal cell necrosis, in bacterial epidermal infections (e.g. impetigo) usually at the edge of a pustule, and less commonly in conditions such as solar keratosis and epidermal carcinomas where the epidermal cells are abnormal by virtue of dysplasia or dyskeratosis. However, it can be difficult to decide whether the epidermal cell abnormalities preceded or followed the onset of the acantholytic process, hence the importance of biopsying an early lesion.

Reticular epidermal degeneration

Ballooning degeneration describes the cytological change seen in epidermal cells infected by some viruses (mainly herpes). The cells become swollen, probably as a result of intracytoplasmic oedema, and the cytoplasm becomes pale; the nucleus may contain a viral inclusion. Similar cytological changes, but without the viral inclusions, may also be seen in some acute skin reactions, particularly drug reactions, and in severe erythema multiforme (see Figs. 8.7 and 14.4(c)). Rupture of the swollen cells releases fluid into the epidermis to produce vesicles or bullae. At an early stage, before adjacent fluid accumulations have merged to become confluent, this mechanism of production of the vesicles is obvious histologically; multiple locules of fluid, associated with some epithelial cells showing ballooning degeneration, are separated from each other by thin septa which are the residue of exploded epithelial cells. This pattern of epidermal destruction is called *reticular degeneration* and, when seen with ballooning change, is usually indicative of viral infection. It may also be seen, in association with spongiosis, in some cases of acute dermatitis. In established viral blisters, some evidence of reticular epidermal degeneration and ballooning of epidermal cells can usually be seen at the edge of the blister. From a histological diagnostic aspect, this pattern of blister formation is the simplest to identify because almost all are of viral cause, and viral inclusions are easily seen at whatever stage the biopsy is performed. Secondary pustular change (e.g. in varicella) may occur but is generally rare in this group of blisters.

Levels of separation in intra-epidermal blisters

Intra-epidermal blisters can be further classified according to the layer in which separation originates:

Subcorneal region

Fluid accumulations beneath the corneal layer are usually packed with neutrophils and are therefore pustules. Causes of subcorneal pustules are impetigo (see Fig. 10.9), some fungal infections, pustular psoriasis and subcorneal pustular dermatosis (see Fig. 8.2).

In prickle cell layer

This is the typical site of the origin of blisters arising by spongiosis and reticular epidermal degeneration, and hence is seen in viral infections (especially herpes/varicella) and in many types of acute and subacute dermatitis.

Suprabasal region

Blisters arising as a result of primary acantholysis (e.g. pemphigus vulgaris and benign familial pemphigus) almost invariably begin in the suprabasal zone, splitting the basal layer (which remains attached to the basal lamina) from the overlying stratum Malpighii which, with the granular and keratin layer, forms the roof of the blister.

Table 8.1 Histological classification of intra-epidermal blisters

Level of separation	Pathological mechanism	Examples
Subcorneal	Spongiotic	Most common; pustules frequent e.g. impetigo
	Acantholytic	Rare; e.g. pemphigus foliaceus
	Reticular degeneration	Rare
Prickle cell layer	Spongiotic	Common; acute and subacute dermatitis
	Acantholytic	Rare; e.g. benign familial pemphigoid
	Reticular degeneration	Common; usually viral e.g. herpes, varicella
Suprabasal	Spongiotic	Rare
	Acantholytic	Common; e.g. pemphigus vulgaris
	Reticular degeneration	Rare

PATTERNS OF INTRA-EPIDERMAL BLISTER FORMATION

Spongiotic blisters

The most common types of spongiotic vesicobullous disorders are those which occur as acute and subacute dermatitis of various causes. These are mainly discussed and illustrated in Chapter 5.

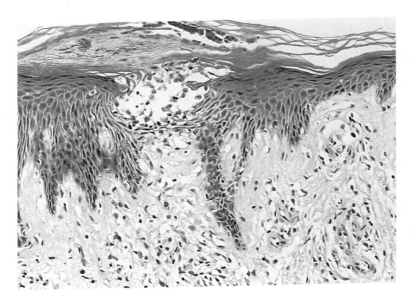

Fig. 8.1. Spongiotic vesicular dermatitis
The epidermis shows early vesicle formation secondary to focal areas of spongiosis; the intercellular oedema can be seen particularly clearly at the edges of the vesicle. The spongiosis and vesicle formation has led to localized expansion of the epidermis and there is overlying parakeratosis. There is a scanty infiltrate of inflammatory cells (in this case, mainly lymphocytes), into the epidermis from the underlying papillary dermis (exocytosis) and this infiltrate is most prominent in the areas where spongiosis and vesiculation are taking place. A few inflammatory cells are present in the fluid of the vesicle. Note that the vesicle is forming in the prickle cell layer.

Fig. 8.2 Spongiotic pustular lesions
Many causes of spongiotic pustular lesions are infective, and these are dealt with in Chapter 10; such causes include impetigo (see Fig. 10.9), septicaemic blisters (see Fig. 10.13) and pustular lesions associated with some fungal infections. Pustule formation is sometimes a feature of psoriasis (see Fig. 6.3). The example illustrated here is the condition of unknown aetiology called descriptively, *subcorneal pustular dermatosis*. This a rare disease characterized by crops of grouped, flaccid pustules, 2–3 mm in diameter, mainly involving the trunk and flexures.

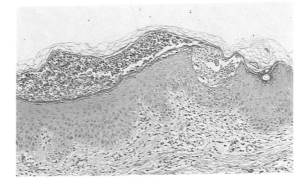

Histologically, there is usually an extensive subcorneal pustule, roofed by a thin, intact corneal layer of keratin. The pustule is usually tense, and packed with neutrophils with few other cell types present. The floor and sides of the pustule are usually clearly defined and there is rarely secondary acantholysis. The upper dermis beneath and surrounding the pustule shows a moderate-to-heavy infiltrate of neutrophils and lymphocytes, with variable numbers of eosinophils. This dermal inflammatory infiltrate is particularly concentrated around prominent and dilated capillaries in the papillary dermis. Strangely, the epidermis wedged between the inflamed dermis below, and the well-formed pustule above, rarely shows a heavy neutrophil infiltrate, and even the spongiosis is often low key. In fact, should a neutrophil infiltrate be prominent in the intervening epidermis, particularly if the neutrophils are grouped, then the diagnosis of a pustular variant of psoriasis should be considered (see Fig. 6.3). The heavy inflammatory dermal infiltrate is the basis of the erythema which precedes pustule formation, and which persists as an expanding rim as the pustule enlarges.

Acantholytic blisters

Most acantholytic blisters originate in the suprabasal region; this is particularly obvious in pemphigus vulgaris, where the separation is usually clean. It is less obvious in benign familial pemphigus, where the acantholytic process also involves cells of the lower half of the prickle cell layer.

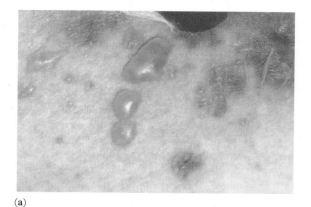

(a)

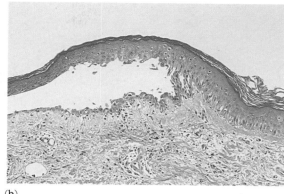

(b)

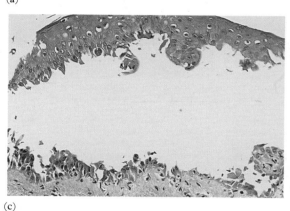

(c)

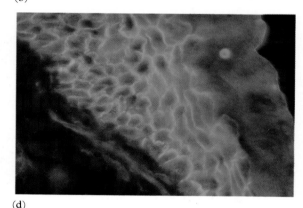

(d)

Fig. 8.3(a)–(d). Pemphigus vulgaris

Clinically, this disease is characterized by flaccid bullae usually appearing on erythematous skin. The bullae contain clear fluid and rupture to produce large erosions (a); lesions are most common on the limbs and flexures (because of friction) and on the trunk and mucosae.

In an established lesion of pemphigus vulgaris, a flaccid bulla is formed as a result of complete separation of the upper epidermal layers from the basal layer, which remains roughly intact and adherent to the basal lamina (b). The cells of the basal layer show incomplete acantholytic separation one from the other such that narrow regular spaces occur between adjacent basal cells, giving rise to the rather fanciful simile of 'rows of tombstones' (c). This suprabasal acantholytic splitting also extends part of the way down skin appendages such as hair follicles. There may be a few scattered acantholytic cells still partly attached to the basal layer. The roof of the flaccid blister is formed of the remaining layers of the epidermis, with a few acantholytic cells partly attached to the lower surface. The blister contains small amounts of low-protein fluid in which are floating a few free acantholytic cells, although inflammatory cells are almost completely absent (but see pemphigus vegetans p. 60). There may be a sparse lymphohistiocytic infiltrate in the upper dermis.

In the very early lesions of pemphigus vulgaris, before the establishment of a blister, separation of the upper surface of the basal cells from the lower surface of the deepest row of the prickle cell layer can easily be seen, as can a lesser degree of separation between the lateral walls of adjacent basal cells. This resembles a particularly uniform and regimented pattern of spongiosis, but is not a truly spongiotic change; rarely a few eosinophils may be present in the lower half of the epidermis where the separation is occurring. It is confusing to call this eosinophilic spongiosis since it detracts from the acantholytic nature of the process.

In old lesions, the intact but partly acantholytic basal layer is progressively replaced by reparative epithelium which slowly thickens and stratifies into the normal epidermal layers. The histological diagnosis at this stage may depend on the demonstration of persisting acantholytic suprabasal splitting in hair follicles, and the presence of some acantholytic cells hanging from the roof of the blister.

Figure 8.3(d) shows the characteristic distribution of IgG in the intercellular spaces of the epidermis in pemphigus vulgaris; IgA, IgM and C3 may be present in a similar distribution. This direct immunofluorescence testing of biopsy skin is an important diagnostic feature in pemphigus vulgaris; it is more sensitive and reliable than the indirect immunofluorescence method using guinea pig oesophagus and patients' serum.

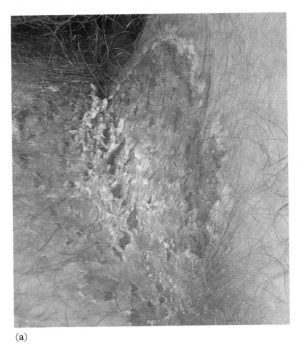

(a)

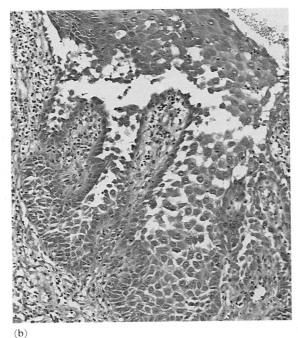

(b)

Fig. 8.4(a) & (b). Benign familial pemphigus

This disease is inherited as an autosomal dominant, but may not present until adulthood. The clinical features are persistent, predominantly flexural, erosions which wax and wane; the surface epidermis has a characteristic rippled appearance, due to the presence of very small vesicles on a rather erythematous base, as seen in the axilla in (a). The vesicles are not true vesicles and have a thick 'roof', as seen in micrograph (b). The lesions are due to defective cell-to-cell adhesion and numbers of desmosomes are reduced. Lesions are usually localized and well-demarcated.

Histologically, this is again a lesion in which blister formation is associated with primary acantholytic separation of epidermal cells, the separation occurring mainly at the junction between basal cells and the lowest layer of prickle cell layer. In this it is similar to pemphigus vulgaris, but there are a number of important histological differences which distinguish them. In benign familial pemphigus the areas of acantholysis are numerous, focal and separated from each other by entirely normal epidermis; they are rarely extensive or confluent and in most cases give rise only to vesicles rather than bullae. The acantholysis is not confined to the suprabasal area, but also involves much of the associated prickle cell layer and may occasionally be almost full thickness as in micrograph (b). There is usually a quite heavy mixed inflammatory cell infiltrate in the upper dermis, the basis of the erythema seen clinically. A final important point is the lack of acantholytic separation in skin appendages such as hair follicles, etc.; when an inappropriately large vesicobullous lesion in benign familial pemphigus has been biopsied, this latter point is a most useful distinguishing feature from pemphigus vulgaris where skin appendage involvement is almost invariable in established bullae. Also, the roof of a bulla in this disease is rarely as crisply defined as in pemphigus vulgaris, mainly because of the extensive involvement of the prickle cell layer in the acantholytic disruptive process; thus, instead of just occasional acantholytic cells in the region of the roof, there are, in benign familial pemphigus, cascades of them, an appearance which has been likened to a crumbling brick wall. Familial benign pemphigus does not show the immunofluorescence changes seen in pemphigus vulgaris.

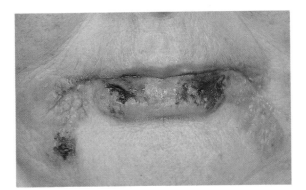

Fig. 8.5. Pemphigus vegetans

This is a rare disorder in which there is blistering and mucosal erosion. However, healing is associated with warty granulations, especially at the corners of the mouth and in flexures. In its early stages it is clinically very like pemphigus vulgaris. Histologically, there is considerable thickening and downgrowth of the hyperplastic epidermis which contains abscesses packed with eosinophils and some free acantholytic cells; the papillary dermis is markedly oedematous and clubbed. Within such a lesion, suprabasal clefting following acantholytic dissociation can usually be found.

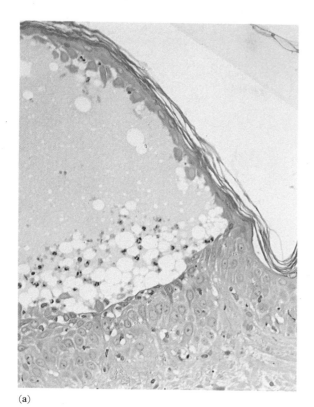

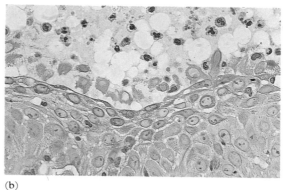

Fig. 8.6(a) & (b). Pemphigus foliaceus (and pemphigus erythematosus)

These usually originate as a persistent but spreading scaly erythema in which superficial flaccid bullae arise. In pemphigus foliaceus lesions may be very widespread, whereas in pemphigus erythematosus they are localized to the face and trunk. In both, bullous lesions may rupture early leaving crusted erosions, and the diseases may be difficult to recognise; shearing of uninvolved skin (Nikolsky's sign) is present. Histologically, the bullae are subcorneal and are characterized by the presence of acantholytic cells in the base, walls and roof of the bulla, as seen in micrographs (a) and (b). Neutrophils may be present in small numbers; rarely are they numerous enough to produce a subcorneal pustule similar to that seen in subcorneal pustular dermatosis (see Fig. 8.2).

(a)

(b)

Other acantholytic lesions

Darier's disease as its synonym, keratosis follicularis, implies is characterized by keratotic papules, and is not a blistering disease. It is discussed and illustrated in Chapter 17. *Transient acantholytic dermatosis* (Grover's disease) is a rare disorder presenting as itchy papules which may develop into vesicles, usually on the chest and proximal limbs. The cause is not known. Histologically, the acantholysis may be focal, suprabasal and associated with dyskeratosis (mimicking Darier's disease), suprabasal and associated with a discrete blister (resembling pemphigus vulgaris), predominantly suprabasal but also involving stratum Malpighii (resembling benign familial pemphigus), or subcorneal (resembling pemphigus foliaceus). Serial sections may reveal one or more of the above patterns in the same lesion. To add to the confusion, 'transient' can mean anything from a couple of weeks to many years.

Reticular degeneration blisters

From a practical, histological viewpoint these are usually easy to identify because of the associated ballooning degeneration of many epidermal cells and the frequent presence of intracellular viral inclusions, since most examples are of viral aetiology. Typical viral reticular degeneration blisters are illustrated in Figures 10.1(d), (e)).

All reticular degeneration blisters appear to originate in the prickle cell layer, but many (particularly viral) become so tense, and are accompanied by such severe cell necrosis, that they force their way down to, and beyond, the basal cell layer and the underlying basement membrane, and into the dermis. In a severe late lesion such as this, the site of origin of the blistering process is not apparent; biopsy of an early lesion is essential. This disruption of basement membrane and damage to underlying dermis leads to permanent scarring (pocking) when the acute phase of epidermal damage is completed.

Reticular degeneration blisters may be seen in the early lesions of some forms of severe erythema multiforme. An example is included here for illustrational purposes; this condition is discussed and illustrated in more detail in Chapter 14.

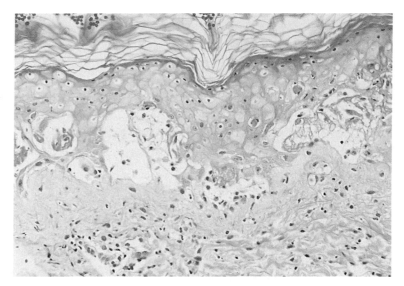

Fig. 8.7. Reticular degeneration blister in erythema multiforme
Note how the blister is developing as a result of the confluence of a number of smaller fluid accumulations, which have themselves resulted from breakdown of clumps of epidermal cells which are immensely swollen by intracellular oedema. Remnants of intact cell membrane form narrow septa between adjacent fluid accumulations. Occasional cells showing ballooning degeneration (but devoid of viral inclusions) are present at the edge of the developing blister.

BASAL BLISTERS

In many cases, blisters originate at the base of the epidermis, in and around the dermo-epidermal junction. For the purposes of this attempt to subdivide blisters, we include the layer of basal cells in this group, since some of the bullous lesions that we classify as basal are a consequence of inflammatory destruction of the basal cell layer with excessive fluid exudation, e.g. bullous lichen planus, bullous lupus erythematosus lesions.

Except in extremely early lesions, it is often not apparent where the initial separation occurred, particularly since so many basal blisters are associated with destructive inflammatory changes around the dermo-epidermal junction. Even if the field were clear for detailed histological examination, and if the very earliest lesion were available, the zone of origin is so narrow that it may be impossible by routine light microscopy to determine whether the separation occurred by splitting through the basal cells, by separation at the deepest cell membrane of the basal cells and the hemidesmosomes tethering them to the basal lamina, the basal lamina itself, or the fibrils anchoring the epidermal basal lamina to the underlying papillary dermis.

High resolution light microscopy using resin-embedded tissues sectioned at 0.5 µm–1 µm may reveal the site of separation, particularly epoxy-resin sections stained with Toluidine Blue. Often the answer is only revealed on electron microscopy, and this is a vital tool in the distinction between the various types of epidermolysis bullosa (see Fig. 8.8). The processes producing intra-epidermal blisters are not applicable to basal blisters. The nature of the associated inflammatory cell infiltrate within the blister and in adjacent epidermis and dermis may provide useful clues to the likely cause, although there are many exceptions to the generalizations below.

Table 8.2 Classification of basal blisters

Predominant inflammatory cell	Important examples
Acellular or scanty	Epidermolysis bullosa, shearing blisters Porphyria cutanea tarda
Eosinophils	Bullous pemphigoid Herpes gestationis
Neutrophils	Dermatitis herpetiformis
Lymphocytes	Bullous lichen planus Bullous lupus erythematosus Blistering erythema multiforme

Basal blisters with minimal inflammatory cell infiltrate

Friction and suction blisters, blistering due to partial thickness burns, and blisters in porphyria cutanea tarda, occur at the basal region and are not accompanied by significant cellular infiltration. The most important disorders in this category are the mechanobullous disorders, e.g. epidermolysis bullosa. Precise histological diagnosis of the various types of epidermolysis bullosa requires the biopsy to show only the earliest stages of separation prior to blister formation; as soon as the blister is developed the precise level of splitting in the basal region may be obscured by secondary tracking of blister fluid and by pressure necrosis. Only at the edge of a blister, and then only when small, is there a chance of the precise localization of early separation being detectable. The situation is further complicated by the fact that electron microscopy is usually essential for accurate diagnosis. In this group of disorders, it is advisable to take two biopsy samples, both of which should be placed in a fixative suitable for high resolution electron microscopy, for example 4% glutaraldehyde. The first sample should be the smallest, most recently developed blister; the other should be from a marked area of skin which has been firmly rubbed with a narrow-pointed but blunt metal instrument, about 30 minutes before the biopsy sample is removed. This mechanical trauma induces early separation facilitating accurate ultrastructural diagnosis and typing. The level of separation in the various types of epidermolysis bullosa is illustrated in the line diagram in Figure 8.8.

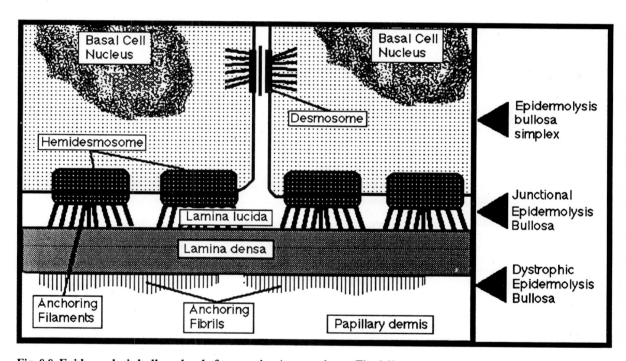

Fig. 8.8. Epidermolysis bullosa: level of separation (see caption to Fig. 8.9)

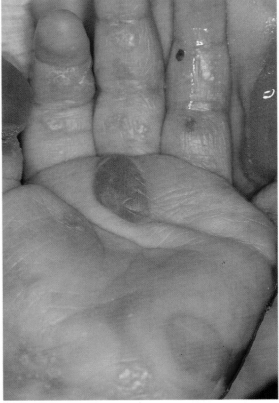

(a)

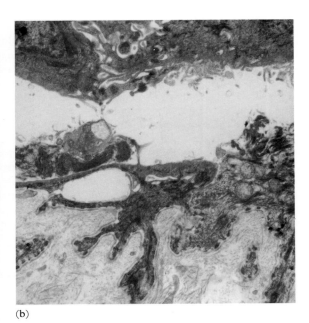

(b)

Fig. 8.9(a) & (b). Epidermolysis bullosa simplex

The clinical characteristics of this condition are determined largely by the level at which the separation occurs in the skin. In the dominantly inherited simplex form where separation originates within the epidermis, blistering heals quickly without scarring or involvement of mucosal surfaces. In junctional forms of the disease, the split occurs through the basement membrane of the skin, so blistering heals without scarring unless there is secondary infection. In the dystrophic form, there is separation below the active dermo-epidermal junction, leading to severe cutaneous and mucosal blistering, followed by scarring and destruction of appendages. Whilst detailed clinical description of the different types of epidermolysis bullosa is beyond the scope of this atlas, one point is worth emphasising; biopsy is essential to make the correct diagnosis, as the phenotype is a poor guide to genotype, especially in severe disease.

The electron micrograph is from a piece of skin which had been traumatized 30 min before biopsy. Note that separation is occurring in the basal cell cytoplasm, leaving the deep basal cell membrane, lamina lucida, anchoring filaments, basal lamina and sublaminal anchoring fibres intact. This permits healing without scarring. This pattern of early separation is characteristic of the simplex variant of epidermolysis bullosa.

Basal blisters with predominant eosinophil infiltrate

Numerous eosinophils are present in association with basal blisters in a small number of clearly defined conditions, particularly bullous pemphigoid and herpes gestationis. The eosinophils are usually present in the upper dermis beneath the blister, in the epidermis at the edge of the blister, and floating free within the blister fluid. There is an admixture of neutrophils and lymphocytes in almost all cases.

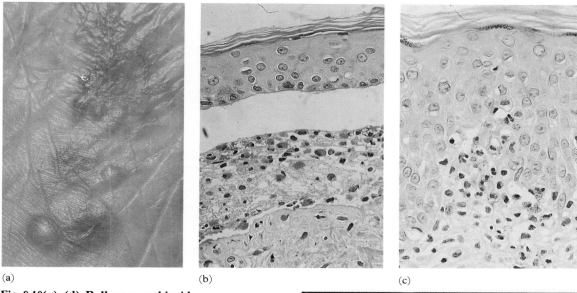

(a)   (b)   (c)

Fig. 8.10(a)–(d). Bullous pemphigoid

This is a disease of the elderly, usually self-limiting, which presents as itchy, urticated red plaques on trunk and limbs, within which tense fluid or blood-filled blisters, often 2–5 cm in size, develop, as seen in (a). Mucosal involvement is uncommon.

Histologically, there is a basal blister, the floor of which is apparently formed by dermal papillae, although most of the basement membrane is intact. The roof of the established blister is therefore formed by the full thickness of the epidermis. The blister contains proteinaceous fluid, threads of fibrin, and eosinophil and neutrophil polymorphs, with the former predominating, as in (b). There is also a heavy mixed inflammatory cell infiltrate in the underlying oedematous dermis; again eosinophils predominate, but lymphocytes and histiocytes may also be numerous. Eosinophils may be present scattered sparsely through the non-blistered epidermis at the rim of the blister, and eosinophil accumulations may occupy the tips of the dermal papillae adjacent to the blister. The most characteristic and diagnostically valuable changes are seen in the skin in which blisters have not yet fully formed. Before full separation of the epidermis, the tips of the dermal papillae become packed with eosinophils, a few of which migrate into the overlying epidermis and appear to discharge their granules, as in (c); at this stage a narrow gap can be seen between the swollen and infiltrated dermal papilla and the overlying epidermis. If the biopsy is taken from erythematous skin, there is usually a significant infiltrate of eosinophils and neutrophils, with a few lymphocytes, mast cells and histiocytes in the dermis beneath the papillae; some eosinophils appear to discharge their granules, so free eosinophil granules may be found in clumps between upper dermal collagen fibres. It is at this

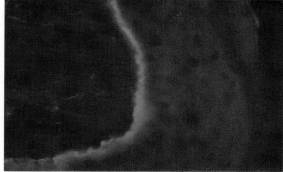

(d)

stage, before a substantial bulla has formed, that a skin biopsy shows most of the diagnostic features, particularly if taken from erythematous skin. In older, established bullae, the basal origin may not be apparent since re-epithelialization of the floor of the bulla can be rapid; furthermore, the epidermis forming the roof of the bulla may undergo necrosis leaving only a horny layer and this, with the re-establishment of epidermal cells on the floor, may give the erroneous impression that the bulla is subcorneal. Rarely, pemphigoid may show almost no inflammatory cell infiltrate, either in bullae or in underlying dermis.

Direct immunofluorescence of the erythematous skin adjacent to the blister shows linear deposition of IgG or C3, as seen in (d), or both, confined to the basement membrane at the intact dermo-epidermal junction; IgA and IgM may also be present in some cases.

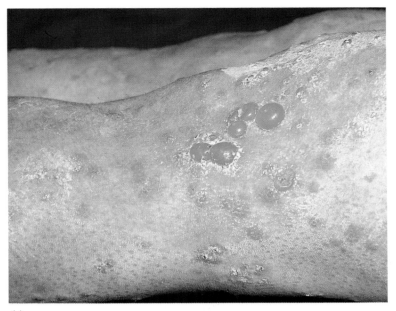

(a)

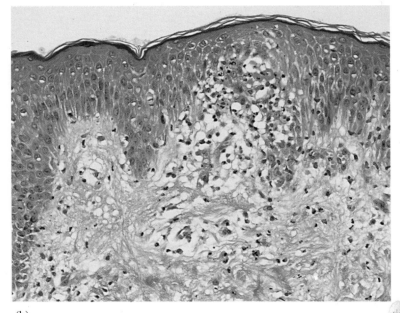

(b)

Fig. 8.11(a) & (b). Herpes gestationis

Lesions usually develop in the second or third trimester of pregnancy as urticated papules or plaques which then blister: they are commonest on the abdomen, and mucosal involvement is rare. The lesions are very similar to those in pemphigoid (a). Neonatal involvement with urticated or bullous lesions can occur, and there is an increased incidence of small-for-dates babies.

Histologically, herpes gestationis shares many features with pemphigoid. Again there may be eosinophilic aggregations at the tips of the oedematous dermal papillae (b), with the formation of a subepidermal blister; there is usually a moderate mixed infiltrate of eosinophils, lymphocytes and histiocytes in the upper dermis, particularly around vessels. Oedema of the dermal papillae is usually marked, and there may be focal necrosis of basal cells leading to the presence of occasional colloid or Civatte bodies. Above such regions of basal cell damage, the epidermis may show spongiosis. Direct immunofluorescence always shows linear deposition of C3 in the basement membrane at the dermo-epidermal junction, and IgG may also be present.

Basal blisters with a predominant neutrophil infiltrate

Neutrophils predominate in dermatitis herpetiformis in the early lesion. Later there is an admixture of eosinophils, and in an established blister it is often impossible to distinguish from bullous pemphigoid on the nature of the cellular infiltrate alone.

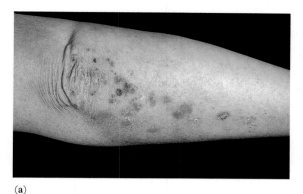

(a)

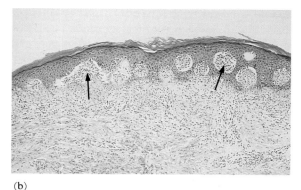

(b)

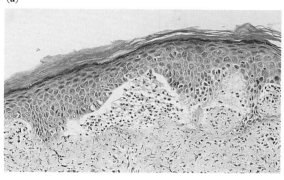

(c)

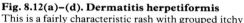

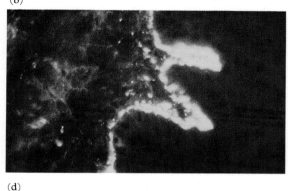

(d)

Fig. 8.12(a)–(d). Dermatitis herpetiformis

This is a fairly characteristic rash with grouped itchy vesicles, usually 4–5 mm across, on the neck, elbows, knees, and sacrum. The vesicles often develop on a base of erythema and urticated papules or plaques, as seen in (a): it usually begins in the 2nd–4th decade.

The diagnostic histological features are best seen in affected erythematous skin in which no substantial vesicles have yet formed. The most significant finding is the presence of accumulations of tightly packed neutrophils at the tips of some dermal papillae (papillary microabscesses), as arrowed in (b), which may also show some fibrin and pyknotic nuclear dust. As the papillary microabscesses enlarge (c), the entire thickness of the overlying epidermis can be seen to be lifting off the damaged papilla, even in skin which is clinically devoid of blisters, and the space becomes occupied by fluid in which a few neutrophils are floating. This change is multifocal and gives rise to a series of minute vesicles which may enlarge by fusion of adjacent lesions. The upper dermis is almost always heavily infiltrated by a mixed inflammatory cell population; in the early stages it is mainly neutrophils, lymphocytes and

histiocytes with occasional eosinophils. With the passage of time, the number of eosinophils increases so that by the time a bulla is apparent clinically, eosinophils may be very numerous, in the upper dermis and in the blister fluid. Nevertheless, neutrophils are still in the majority, unlike in bullous pemphigoid. This again emphasizes the importance of biopsy of an early erythematous lesion, rather than an established bulla.

Direct immunofluorescence shows characteristic deposition of IgA in a granular, clumped pattern at the tips of the dermal papillae in non-lesional and erythematous non-blistering skin. This is absent at a late stage of papillary destruction when the basal blister has formed.

Linear IgA disease (bullous dermatosis of childhood) shows clinical features and some of the histological changes similar to those seen in dermatitis herpetiformis. Bullae on an erythematous base is a common feature and may be symmetrical. Immunofluorescence shows linear deposition of IgA at the basement membrane without the concentration at the papillary tips seen in dermatitis herpetiformis.

Basal blistering with a predominantly neutrophil infiltrate may be seen in *acute bacterial cellulitis*, but this is obvious clinically and is distinct because of the heavy neutrophil infiltrate and oedema in all layers of the dermis and upper subcutis; the epidermal blistering is a secondary phenomenon. Basal blisters may also form in some cases of *acute and subacute lupus erythematosus*, and is associated with a local area of severe upper dermal oedema, active hydropic degeneration and necrosis of cells of the basal layer, and fibrinoid necrosis of upper dermal collagen with a variable neutrophil infiltrate (see Chapter 9).

Basal blisters with a predominantly lymphohistiocytic infiltrate

Basal blistering, leading to bulla formation, is an occasional feature of lichen planus; this is discussed in Chapter 7. Blister formation is a result of destruction of the basal layer associated with excessive fluid accumulation. The floor of the ulcer is formed by naked dermis which usually shows the dense, band-like lymphocytic infiltrate characteristic of lichen planus, and lymphocytes spill into the blister fluid; at the edge of the blister, typical histological features of lichen planus can usually be seen (see Fig. 8.1). Blisters with a scanty lymphohistiocytic infiltrate may also form in some cases of subacute or chronic lupus erythematosus as a consequence of basal layer destruction, the lymphocytes representing spill-over from the usual upper dermal chronic inflammatory cell infiltrate. Another disease in which basal (sub-epidermal) blisters may form is erythema multiforme; the macular, papular and blistering lesions in this histologically complex disorder are discussed and illustrated in Chapter 14. Vesicles and bullae may occur superimposed upon the macular and papular lesions, and are usually due to severe oedema of the papillary dermis associated with basal layer hydropic degeneration and necrosis leading to subepidermal separation, the roof of the blister being composed of the entire thickness of the epidermis. The base of the blister is dermis which is usually heavily infiltrated by lymphocytes and histiocytes, some of which appear in the blister fluid.

Diagnosis of blistering and pustular disorders

Despite the broad outlines given above, accurate histological diagnosis of this group of conditions can be difficult. It is vital that only early lesions are biopsied for histological examination; in late lesions the site of origin of a blister may be difficult to define. For example, in a late bullous pemphigoid lesion the reflooring of a bulla by regenerating epithelium may obscure the fact that it was originally a basal blister. In those blisters in which the nature of the associated inflammatory cell infiltrate is of diagnostic value, the picture may become confused in late lesions; for example, in established lesions of dermatitis herpetiformis the late arrival of eosinophils may conceal the fact that in the early, diagnostic stages, the reaction is predominantly neutrophilic. This may lead to an erroneous histological diagnosis of bullous pemphigoid. If the blister or pustule arises on an erythematous base, then some of the erythematous skin should be included in the biopsy sample since this area may show diagnostically important pre-blister changes. In most blistering disorders it is advisable to take an additional biopsy sample, or to divide a large biopsy, so that part can be sent to the laboratory to be snap-frozen for immunofluorescent examination.

Direct immunofluorescent examination of a skin biopsy plays an important complementary role to histology in the diagnosis of the blistering disorders. For successful and consistent results the same precautions should be taken as already described for histological diagnosis. The biopsy should normally be of an early lesion, preferably of the often erythematous skin at the edge of a bulla or vesicle, although non-lesional skin is suitable in dermatitis herpetiformis. An excised skin ellipse is preferable to a punch biopsy since it is easier to handle in the laboratory, but a 4mm or 6mm punch biopsy of skin may be adequate provided that the site is carefully selected. Immunofluorescent techniques are performed on unfixed frozen sections, so the specimen must be sent quickly to the laboratory in an unfixed state for immediate snap-freezing in liquid nitrogen. Drying out of the specimen renders frozen sectioning more difficult, and can produce poor histological results; it can be prevented by folding the skin biopsy in gauze which has been soaked in normal saline then squeezed until just damp.

The identification of the various immunoglobulins and some complement factors, and their site of localisation within the skin, are of considerable diagnostic value, since some blistering diseases have characteristic patterns. Some of these have been illustrated in Figs. 8.3d, 8.10d, and 8.12d, and discussed briefly in the preceding text; they are summarised in Table 8.3 opposite.

Indirect immunofluorescence is of value in the demonstration of circulating intercellular antibodies in the serum of patients of patients with pemphigus. The titre partially reflects the degree of disease activity, so may be low in the early stages of the disease and during remission. The antibody is demonstrable in all patterns of pemphigus, including the vegetans and foliaceous types, and is also present in penicillamine-induced pemphigus.

Many patients with bullous pemphigoid have a circulating basement membrane zone; this may disappear completely during periods of remission.

Finally, where epidermolysis bullosa is suspected, electron microscopy will be necessary to determine the precise type, thus the biopsy sample should be placed in an EM fixative such as glutaraldehyde. The biopsy procedure to be followed in epidermolysis bullosa is described on page 63.

Table 8.3 Immunofluorescence findings in blisters

Disease	Ig's and complements	Localization
Pemphigus vulgaris Pemphigus vegetans Pemphigus foliaceous	} IgG (IgA, IgM, C3)	Intercellular spaces of epidermis (chicken-wire distribution)
Bullous pemphigoid	IgG/C3 (IgA, IgM)	Linear basal lamina
Herpes gestationis	C3, Clq, C4 (IgG)	Linear basal lamina
Dermatitis, herpetiformis	IgA (C3, IgG, IgM)	Granular, along basal lamina especially dermal papillae (non-lesional skin)
IgA bullous dermatosis	IgA (IgG)	Linear basal lamina

9. Lupus erythematosus and other connective tissue disorders

Introduction

Cutaneous involvement in lupus erythematosus, dermatomyositis, systemic sclerosis and polyarteritis is usual. Although some of the physical signs are similar (for instance, livedo reticularis and nail-fold telangiectases), these diseases are usually distinctive. Overlap does occur, leading to such concepts as mixed connective tissue disease, and eosinophilic fasciitis may be an early phase of systemic sclerosis. Not surprisingly, there are also similarities in some of the histological features of these diseases.

Lupus erythematosus

The clinical and histological appearances seen in skin involvement in lupus erythematosus (LE) are variable; however, the two major manifestations, the classical butterfly rash and the chronic discoid lesions, have fairly consistent histological appearances.

Some cutaneous manifestations of lupus fall into neither the butterfly nor discoid categories, and there are other less common patterns which vary in severity, distribution and clinical appearance. These include an erythematous maculopapular eruption which may be photosensitive, mucosal lesions with ulceration, vasculitic lesions with purpura, and red papules which heal to leave atrophic macules. Histologically, these lesions show changes intermediate between acute lupus (butterfly) and chronic discoid; for example, there is usually prominent hydropic basal cell degeneration and upper dermal oedema associated with an inflammatory cell infiltrate greater than that seen in acute LE, but less than in chronic LE. An acute neutrophilic vasculitis affecting superficial small dermal vessels may be seen when there is clinical purpura. Hyperkeratosis (scaling) is usually minimal.

Fig. 9.1(a)–(d). Systemic lupus erythematosus (SLE): butterfly rash (*illustrations opposite*)

This eruption occurs most commonly across the nose and malar regions, and may result from photosensitivity. The lesions are plaques which are raised, scaly and erythematous, with pin-point telangiectasia (a). The raised appearance is partly due to scale, but mainly to dermal oedema (b), whilst the erythema is the result of dilated upper dermal vessels. When upper dermal capillaries are prominently dilated, or if there is some eosinophilic degeneration of vessel walls (c), with extravasation of red cells, the pin-point telangiectasia may be clinically prominent. Both the erythema and telangiectasia are easily visible through the almost invariably thinned epidermis. Variable hyperkeratosis produces irregular scaling. The most significant histological feature of lupus skin lesions is the presence of hydropic degeneration of the basal layer of the epidermis, often associated with the presence of eosinophilic colloid or Civatte bodies (arrowed in c) representing dead basal cells; this feature is also seen in lichen planus (see Fig. 8.1). Figure 9.1(d) shows linear deposition of IgG at the basal lamina demonstrated by direct immunofluorescence of non-lesional light-exposed skin. The intense linear fluorescence at the basal lamina of the epidermis contrasts with the irregular yellow autofluorescence of the collagen fibres in the dermis. This finding is variable, and is therefore unreliable as a diagnostic test.

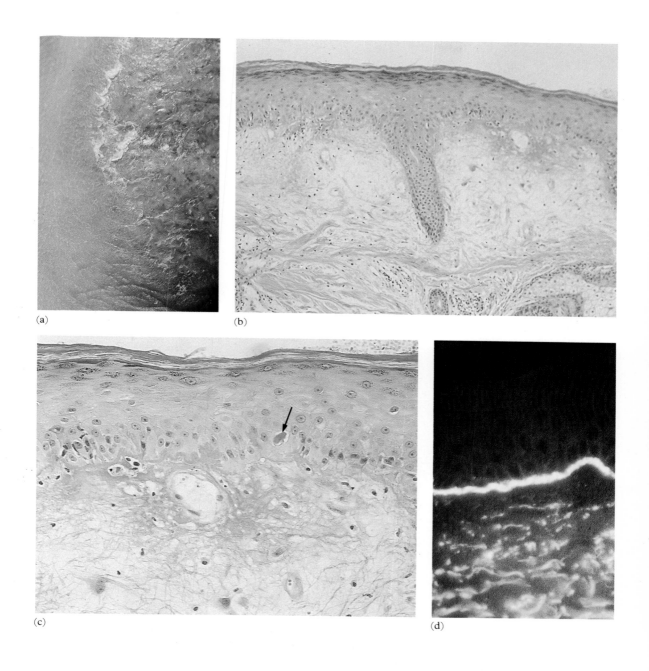

(a)

(b)

(c)

(d)

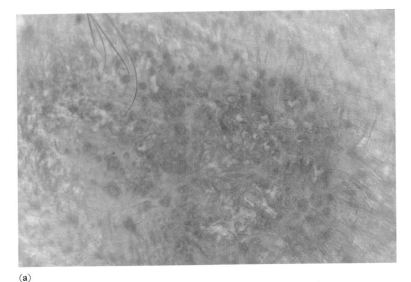

(a)

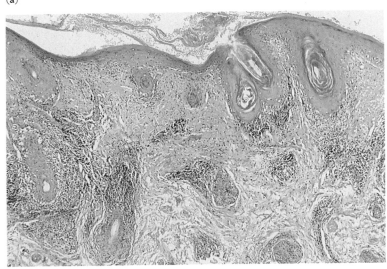

(b)

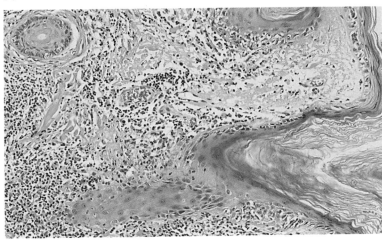

(c)

Fig. 9.2(a), (b) & (c). Chronic discoid lesions in lupus erythematosus (LE)

Lesions occur most commonly on the face, scalp and hands, and produce red, scaly, telangiectatic plaques which heal centrally with atrophy and loss of pigment. Prominent plugging of follicles with keratin is common (a).

The characteristic histological features are: (i) basal cell hydropic degeneration, often with necrosis of scattered basal cells and Civatte body formation (see Fig 4.5); (ii) dermal oedema and telangiectasia, sometimes with red cell extravasation; (iii) variable chronic inflammatory cell infiltrate in the dermis, particularly around blood vessels and skin appendages; (iv) upper dermal fibrosis; (v) epidermal atrophy with hyperkeratosis and follicular plugging with keratin. These features can be seen in micrographs (b) and (c). In very early lesions, the histological changes are similar to those seen in the butterfly rash (see Fig. 9.1), viz. basal cell hydropic degeneration, dermal oedema and telangiectasia. As the lesion ages the dermal oedema is supplemented by increasing lymphocyte infiltration, and the epidermal thinning becomes progressively more apparent, as does the hyperkeratosis producing the scaling, and follicular plugging with keratin. This last feature is particularly prominent in skin rich in hair follicles, e.g. scalp. In old lesions the epidermis is often markedly thinned and the dermis shows fibrous scarring; the inflammatory infiltrate often partially subsides although some persists around hair follicles, where the characteristic basal cell changes can often still be seen (c). Marked follicular plugging with keratin also remains although many hair follicles and other skin appendages are eventually totally destroyed, leaving an atrophic area of alopecia. In active lesions, basal layer destruction leads to fall out of melanin into the dermis where it is phagocytosed by macrophages (melanophages), producing occasional irregular reticulate hyperpigmentation, visible clinically when the erythema subsides. With the passage of time the area becomes hypopigmented, although the melanophages are still present histologically; this is probably the obscuring effect of increasing dermal fibrosis.

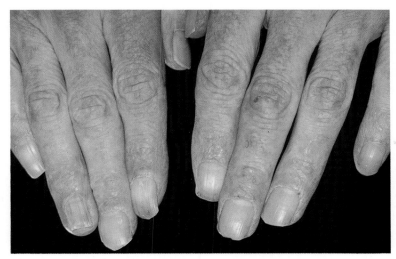

(a)

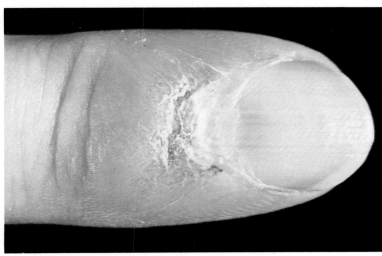

(b)

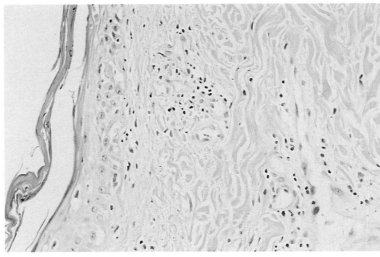

(c)

Fig. 9.3(a), (b) & (c). Skin lesions in dermatomyositis

The rash is variable: characteristically there is purplish erythema involving face, eyelids and extensor surfaces (a), with oedema and scaling. Dilated thrombosed nail-fold capillaries are also characteristic (b), but are seen in other connective tissue disorders as well. Generalized follicular keratosis with alopecia, and livedo (see p. 102) also occur; lesions may subsequently become poikilodermatous (see Fig. 22.6a). Cutaneous manifestations of dermatomyositis can resemble the various patterns of lupus skin involvement, particularly the acute and subacute types.

Histologically, upper dermal oedema, which may be severe, and scanty perivascular inflammatory cell infiltrate are usual features. However, examination of many levels of the biopsy will usually reveal features resembling those of acute lupus (see Fig. 9.1), viz. hydropic basal cell degeneration, with associated inflammatory cell invasion into the lower epidermal layers, focal epidermal atrophy etc. as in (c); distinction from lupus may be difficult. In the lesions which resemble poikiloderma, the basal cell abnormalities are associated with a heavier, more uniform chronic inflammatory cell infiltrate in the upper dermis, resembling the band-like infiltrate seen in lichen planus, with which it may be confused histologically, although the epidermis is usually thinned and shows none of the acanthosis and rete ridge accentuation seen in classical lichen planus (cf. Fig. 7.2). The inflammatory infiltrate becomes more scanty as the lesion ages and increasing numbers of pigment-laden melanophages are present, a measure of the prolonged basal cell destruction.

In summary, the variable histological appearances of the skin in dermatomyositis make skin biopsy unreliable; the diagnosis must usually be based on clinical features, a raised blood creatine phosphokinase level, and an abnormal muscle biopsy.

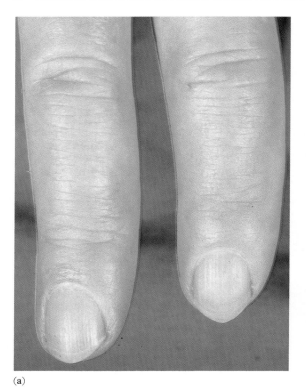

(a)

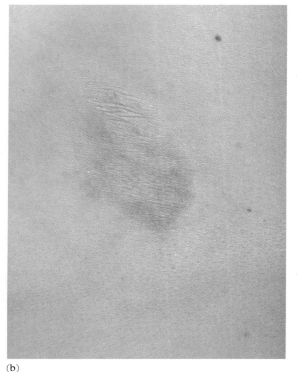

(b)

Fig. 9.4(a), (b) & (c). Scleroderma (generalized and morphoea)

Although these two diseases are probably unrelated, there are close histological similarities. In systemic sclerosis, seen in micrograph (a) there is gradually increasing rigidity, tightening and atrophy of the skin, especially on the fingers and face. Macular telangiectases are common on the face. Morphoea, illustrated in (b), may be localized or diffuse; lesions are initially creamy coloured immobile thickened dermal plaques on the trunk or limbs and have a purplish edge when active. They may become atrophic or depressed, or coalesce to involve large areas. In early lesion of both systemic sclerosis and morphoea, the major abnormality is a chronic inflammatory cell (mainly lymphocytic) infiltrate in the mid- and lower dermis and upper subcutis. This infiltrate is scattered between dermal collagen fibres (which may show dense thickening) and subcutaneous adipocytes, but is often more concentrated around blood vessels and skin appendages in the dermis, and within the interstitial fibrous septae in the subcutis. The epidermis is usually normal, and the papillary dermis is usually minimally involved. With the passage of time, the dermal inflammatory infiltrate becomes less prominent, the collagen of the reticular dermis becomes dense and contracted, and there is progressive collagenization of the upper subcutis (c), which probably accounts for the loss of mobility of the skin. As the dermis and upper subcutis becomes more sclerotic, the skin appendages slowly atrophy

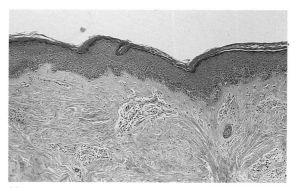

(c)

and largely disappear and the overlying epidermis thins, with flattening of rete ridges. Often the only skin appendage remnants identifiable in the end-stage sclerotic morphoeic lesion are fragments of arrector pili muscle. A single morphoeic plaque may show both early inflammatory and late sclerotic changes if biopsied at an opportune time, when the lesion is well-established but still expanding; the central edge show sclerotic changes whilst the raised expanding edge shows the active inflammatory lesion. It is important that the biopsy should be deep enough in both diseases to include subcutis.

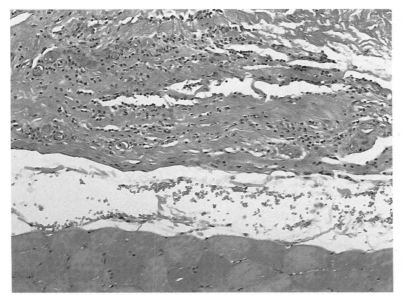

Fig. 9.5. Eosinophilic fasciitis
This presents as acute cutaneous induration of abdomen and limbs, associated with fever, raised erythrocyle sedimentation rate (ESR), peripheral blood eosinophilia and hypergammaglobulinaemia. There are frequently other features of connective tissue disorder such as Raynaud's phenomenon and myositis, and it may progess to systemic sclerosis. Histologically, the diagnosis can only be made with certainly in a substantial biopsy which includes skin, subcutis, fascia and preferably some underlying muscle. The major abnormality is in the fascia which is thickened and homogenous, with extension of strands of fibrous thickening upwards into subcutaneous fat and occasionally downwards into skeletal muscle. There is a variable chronic inflammatory cell infitrate, but eosinophils are usually only numerous when there is a significant blood eosinophilia. This micrograph shows the fascial layer between the subcutis above (not shown) and the skeletal muscle below. The normally thin fascia is thickened and degenerate, and infiltrated by a mixed inflammatory infiltrate in which neutrophils and lymphocytes are numerous, but eosinophils scanty. The underlying skeletal muscle showed a focal myositis (not seen here).

Mixed connective tissue disease (MCTD)

This disease has many of the serological features of systemic lupus erythematosus, but a large percentage of the patients also possess anti-RNP (ribonucleoprotein) antibody. However, the clinical picture differs from classical SLE. There is Raynaud's phenomenon, arthritis, myositis, and dysphagia due to oesophageal involvement; pulmonary involvement with progressive fibrosis is frequent. Skin rashes are rare, and the major cutaneous involvement is Raynaud's phenomenon, although some patients may have a cutaneous lymphocytic vasculitis (see Fig. 12.5) at some stage in the illness.

Other cutaneous manifestations of connective tissue disease

The lesions described above are clinically distinct skin lesions associated with specific connective tissue disorders. The characteristic granulomatous nodules of rheumatoid disease are discussed and illustrated in Figure 11.5, and the vasculitic lesions associated with polyarteritis nodosa and its variants are discussed and illustrated in Chapter 12. It is important to realise that an acute neutrophilic vasculitis may occur in some patterns of systemic lupus erythematosus and in rheumatoid disease. In the latter, the vasculitis may produce characteristic skin ulcers with purple edges indicative of a vasculitic basis. The finding of an unexplained lymphocytic vasculitis histologically should always stimulate serological investigation for an underlying connective tissue disorder (see p. 105).

10. Infections of the skin

Introduction

Skin infections can be classified both by the type of organism involved and whether skin involvement is direct or indirect. In this chapter, the disorders are dealt with according the type of organism involved, with additional notes on indirect effects. They are discussed under the following headings:

1. Viral infections;
2. Bacterial infections;
3. Fungal infections;
4. Protozoal infections;
5. Parasitic infestations.

VIRAL INFECTIONS

Viruses can affect skin *directly* and *indirectly*. The following viruses act directly:

Herpes virus: Varicella-zoster and simplex

Human papilloma virus: Warts due to infection by the human papilloma virus (HPV) are particularly common on the hands and feet in children, but occur elsewhere, e.g. genitalia and mucosal surfaces. Variability in clinical appearance depends largely on the site and the amount of trauma to which they are subjected. Common sites and virus strains are summarized in Table 10.1:

Pox virus: Molluscum contagiosum

Table 10.1 Human papilloma virus types and associated lesions

HPV type	Associated lesion
HPV 1,4	Plantar wart
HPV2	Hand wart
HPV3, 10	Plane warts
HPV 5, 8, 9, 12, 14, 15, 17, 19–29	Epidermodysplasia verruciformis lesions
HPV 6	Laryngeal and genital warts
HPV 16, 18	Genital warts, cervix/penis carcinoma
HPV 30	Laryngeal papillomas

Examples of direct viral infection of skin

Fig. 10.1(a)–(f). Herpes simplex, herpes zoster and varicella *(illustrations opposite)*
The lesions produced by these viruses have many features in common. All produce red macules which develop into vesicles as in chicken pox shown in (a) and then pustules; the vesicles are characteristically thin-walled and easily ruptured, and may be umbilicated. The diseases are distinguished by the rate of development of lesions, which in varicella-zoster can progress from macule to papule to vesicle and finally to pustule in only 12 hours, and also by their distribution. The trunk is mainly involved with scattered lesions in varicella, whilst they are usually confined to a dermatome in zoster (b), and a localized cluster of vesicles in herpes simplex (c).

A typical lesion shows predominantly epidermal abnormalities. A vesicle forms as a result of necrosis of virus-infected epidermal cells which show a characteristic ballooned appearance, being spherical and acantholoytic (d), often showing intranuclear eosinophilic viral inclusions (arrow in (e)). Other epithelial cells are swollen and pale as a result of intracellular oedema. Acantholytic epidermal cells float about in the watery and fibrinous fluid in the vesicles, inflammatory cells being rare except in pustular chicken pox. The dermal changes are variable; there is usually an inflammatory cell infiltrate but occasionally a neutrophilic vasculitis may be seen.

The above changes are seen irrespective of whether the lesions are due to type 1 herpes simplex (non-genital), type 2 (genital) or varicella-zoster (chicken pox and shingles); histological variation is more dependent on the age of the biopsied lesion rather than the virus. Electron micrograph (f) shows the characteristic herpes virus particles (arrow) in a necrotic epidermal cell from a lip lesion of herpes simplex.

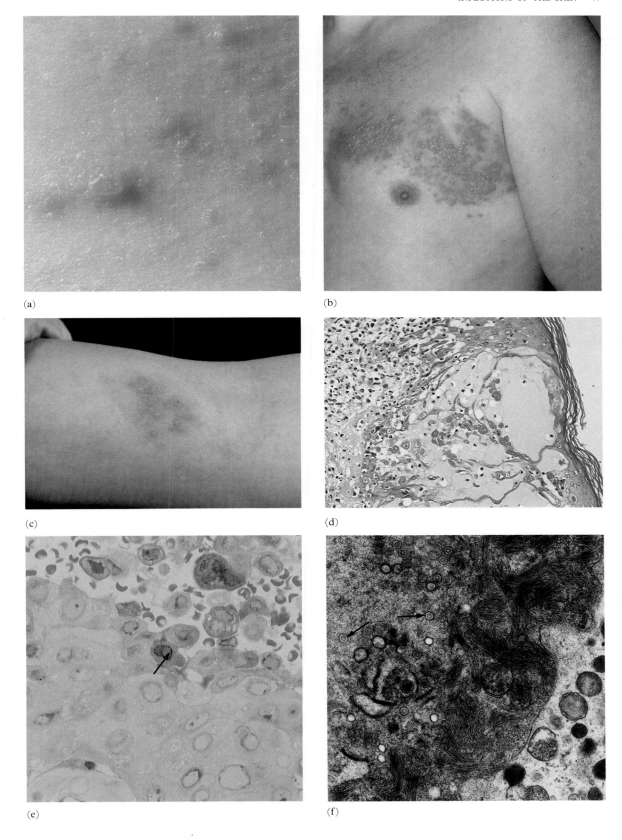

(a)

(b)

(c)

(d)

(e)

(f)

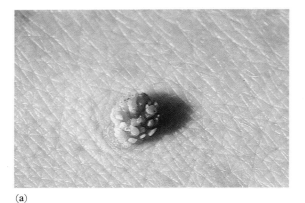

(a)

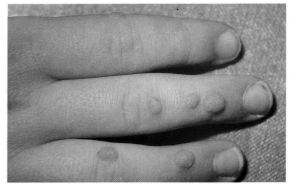

(b)

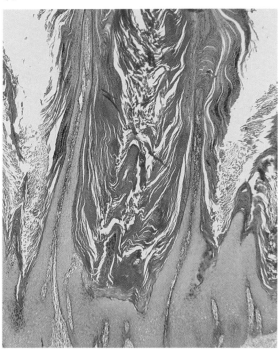

(c)

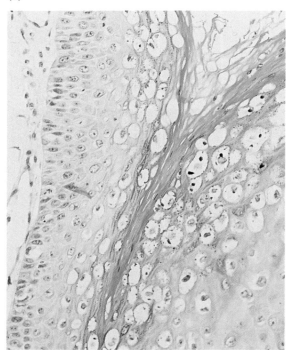

(d)

Fig. 10.2(a)–(d) Verruca vulgaris (common viral wart)

Warts are usually filiform, with fronds arising from a well-circumscribed base and covered by thick keratin, as seen in (a). Such an appearance is likely to be seen on the scalp and oral mucosa, but warts on more exposed areas such as the hands and knees tend to be traumatized and are less filiform, as in (b), although the surface remains divided due to persistence of the base of the fronds; lesions on the soles are flat. The histological features of these two patterns are essentially the same. The fronds are composed of papillary acanthotic epidermis overlain by hyperkeratosis and, by a characteristic feature, narrow 'spires' of parakeratosis emanating from the frond tips. The rete pegs are thickened and elongated at the edge of the wart, often pointing inwards towards the centre producing the solid thickened base of the wart. Beneath the base there is a variable dermal chronic inflammatory cell infiltrate, particularly heavy in old, chronically traumatized warts, especially those which have become so hyperkeratotic as to form a cutaneous horn (see Fig. 17.7). The thickened epidermis contains many vacuolated cells in the upper prickle cell and granular layers, usually most obvious in the troughs between adjacent fronds. Keratohyaline granules are very numerous and often abnormally large in the granular layer, particularly alongside an area of vacuolated cells.

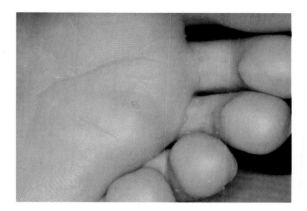

Fig. 10.3 Plantar warts

Plantar warts occur on the sole and are particularly common in children of school age. Occasionally solitary, they are more often multiple in clusters which can coalesce to produce a substantial lesion which may be painful, particularly if situated on the ball or heel of the foot. By the time they are symptomatic, they appear as flat or slightly raised lesions with a pale collar of skin surrounding a rough-surfaced centre showing brown or black spots.

They differ significantly in their histological features from the exophytic warts. The epithelial cells contain large eosinophilic or purplish bodies within the cytoplasm, resembling the molluscum bodies of molluscum contagiosum, but representing abnormal keratohyaline. Some nuclei are large and pale-staining; others are small, round and deeply basophilic, and surrounded by a non-staining halo.

Fig. 10.4(a) & (b) Planar wart (verruca plana)

Plane warts are multiple small, slightly raised elevations usually occurring on the face but can occur in other sites, for example, on the hands. They are normally approximately the same colour as the surrounding skin but can be slightly brownish if hyperkeratosis is a significant feature.

The histological features are characteristic, with acanthosis and varying degrees of hyperkeratosis but with a complete lack of papillomatosis. The overlying keratin is almost always orthokeratotic. Cells showing the features of virus infection (koilocytes) with prominent cytoplasmic vacuolation, are largely confined to the granular layer and the upper layers of the prickle cell layer (b).

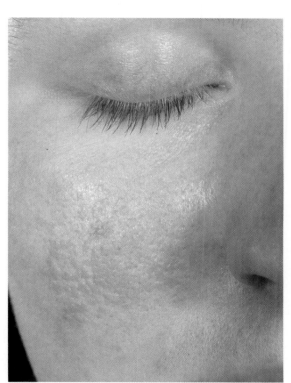

(a)

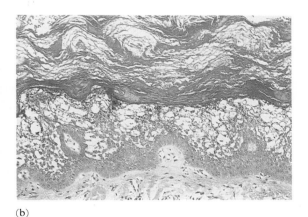

(b)

As the diagnosis is usually obvious, most of the viral warts seen in the pathology department will have been biopsied because they are clinically atypical, and it is not surprising that many are histologically atypical too. They are usually removed to exclude dysplasia or squamous carcinoma. This may be a diagnostic problem for the histologist, but careful examination at a number of levels will usually reveal spikes of parakeratosis and the characteristic vacuolated cells and clumpy keratohyaline. A further trap is the healing viral wart in which the lower layers of the epidermis may show significant mitotic activity and some cellular and nuclear atypia, causing potential confusion with intra-epidermal carcinoma or actinic keratosis; the presence of viral changes in the upper epidermis usually reveals the true nature of the lesion.

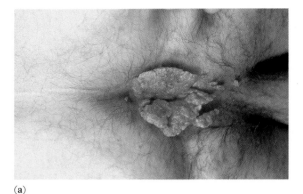

(a)

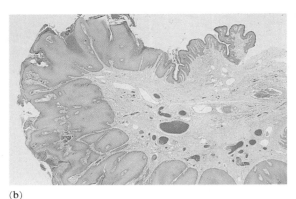

(b)

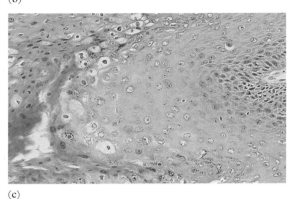

(c)

Fig. 10.5(a), (b) & (c) Condyloma acuminatum (genital warts)

The lesions are fleshy papules and characteristically have a filiform or velvety surface. They are usually grouped around the anus, as in (a), vaginal introitus or shaft of the penis, mainly in sexually active adults. They are strongly associated with the subsequent development of cervical and penile carcinoma when due to HPV types 16 and 18, though there is no proof of a causal relationship.

They are characterized histologically by very prominent acanthosis with elongation and broadening of rete ridges which are often smoothly rounded and sometimes branched, as in (b). The increase in thickness is mainly due to expansion of the prickle cell layer, some of the cells of which are vacuolated and may show perinuclear halos, as in (c). There is an increase in cells in mitosis and this feature, taken with the large branching rete ridges, may lead to confusion with the verrucous type of squamous carcinoma.

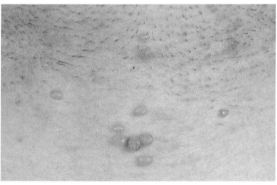

(a)

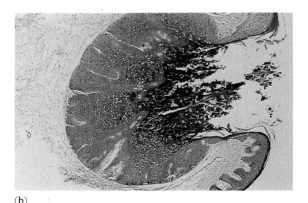

(b)

Fig. 10.6(a) & (b) Molluscum contagiosum

These are common in children and usually appear on the trunk or face as a group of whitish domed papules, 1–5 mm in diameter (a). Characteristically, the lesions develop a central core as they enlarge, from which granular material can be expressed when they are squeezed.

Histologically, the appearances are absolutely characteristic. The epidermis extends down into the dermis in small rounded lobules with a clearly defined lower edge; a cluster of adjacent lobules produces the clinically apparent nodule, as seen in (b). The epidermis is thickened and histologically abnormal, and the central area contains a plug of keratin in which numerous molluscum bodies are present.

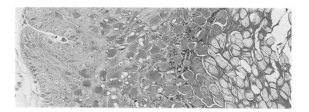

Fig. 10.7 Molluscum bodies
In the cytoplasm of the spinous keratinocytes immediately above the basal layer are small eosinophilic viral inclusions; these become large and more numerous in more superficial epidermal cells until they occupy most of the cytoplasm near the granular layer. As they enlarge, they become progressively more basophilic, and in the horny layer, appear as large, basophilic, rounded masses called molluscum bodies.

Indirect effects of viruses on skin

Viruses can affect the skin indirectly and cause a characteristic exanthem. More often, the appearance is an erythematous, macular, papular rash or blotchy erythema. This is called toxic erythema, and may also accompany bacterial infections or be a manifestation of a drug reaction (see Ch. 14). The histological appearances of a toxic erythema are fairly constant, and give no clue to its cause; there is dilatation of small blood vessels in the upper and mid-dermis, with a dense lymphocytic infiltrate closely applied around them. At present, HIV virus has not been identified in the skin lesions of AIDS, and it is likely that the effect of HIV on skin is indirect. Many patients with AIDS develop infective skin lesions, and widespread molluscum contagiosum and severe herpes simplex can occur. Oral hairy leukoplakia in AIDS is probably due to mucosal infection with Epstein-Barr virus.

The common condition, *pityriasis rosea* (see Fig. 2.2(a)) may have a viral aetiology, but the evidence is insubstantial.

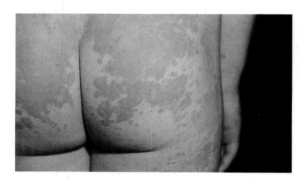

Fig. 10.8 Viral-induced erythema
The clinical photograph shows typical indirect effect of viruses on the skin. There is a toxic erythema, in this case producing a characteristic lesion on the buttocks, the so-called 'slapped cheek syndrome'; this is commonly associated with a parvovirus infection.

BACTERIAL INFECTIONS

Table 10.2   Simple classification of bacterial skin infections

Staphylococcal	Impetigo and ecthyma Folliculitis, 'scalded skin' syndrome
Streptococcal	Some impetigo and ecthyma Celluitis, erysipelas
Neisseria	Acute and chronic gonococcaemia Acute and chronic meningococcaemia
Mycobacterial	Tuberculosis Leprosy Atypical mycobacteria
Treponema	*T. pallidum*—syphilis *T. pertenue*—yaws *T. carateum*—pinta
Corynebacterium	Erythrasma
Erysipelothrix	Erysipeloid

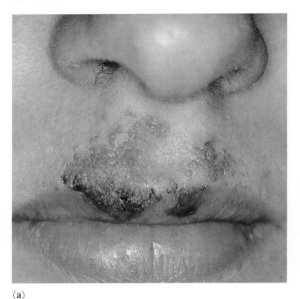

(a)

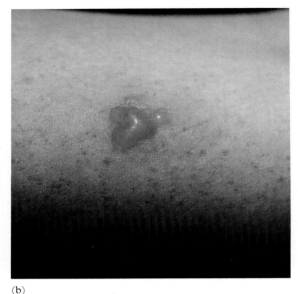

(b)

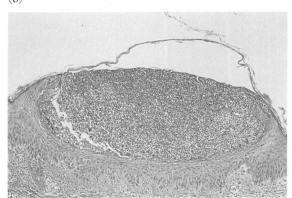

(c)

Fig. 10.9(a), (b) & (c) Impetigo
This is common in children, and lesions enlarge and spread
quickly. They may be small vesicles which quickly rupture
and form plaques with a characteristic yellow crust, as seen
in (a), or large flaccid bullae which initially contain serous
fluid, as seen in (b), and subsequently pus. Lesions are often
widespread, usually involving the face, trunk and limbs.
The type of lesion seems to be determined by the organism;
crusted plaques are usually associated with staphylococci
and streptococci, whilst bullous impetigo is probably due to
local production of a staphylococcal epidermolytic toxin. In
infants this may cause large, rapidly spreading, tender
erythematous areas with erosions and cleavage of the
epidermis in the granular cell layer (pemphigus
neonatorum); systemic, rather than local, distribution of the
toxin results in the widespread severe tender erythema and
blistering of the 'staphylococcal scalded skin syndrome'.

The most obvious lesion in impetigo is the pustule in
the upper layers of the epidermis, in the region of the
granular layer, as in (c). The pustule contains numerous
neutrophil polymorphs, a little fluid and some Gram-
positive cocci which, if numerous, can occasionally be
demonstrated in a paraffin section by a Gram stain. The
remaining layers of the epidermis beneath the pustule show
variable spongiosis and neutrophilic infiltration; where
spongiosis is marked there may be a few free-floating
acantholytic epidermal cells. There is a mixed neutrophil
and lymphocyte infiltrate in the upper dermis, usually focal
and confined to the area beneath a pustule. In *bullous
impetigo* the changes differ, in that a bulla forms in the same
location in the upper epidermis instead of a pustule,
neutrophils being almost entirely absent from the
epidermis; however, there is usually a mixed neutrophil and
lymphocyte infiltrate in the upper dermis beneath the bulla.
In the staphylococcal scalded skin syndrome, extensive
blisters form in the subcorneal region of the epidermis such
that the roof of the blister is composed of stratum corneum
only. The underlying epidermis is usually mildly acanthotic
and there may be focal spongiosis. The blister contains
proteinaceous fluid, a few neutrophils and occasional
acantholytic squamous cells, particularly at the blister base
and periphery. The dermis shows a mixed inflammatory cell
infiltrate, including some neutrophils.

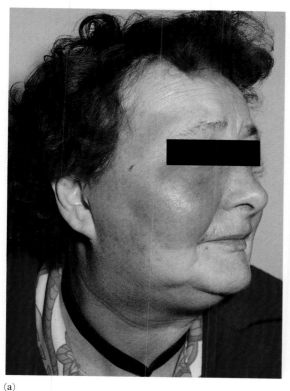

(a)

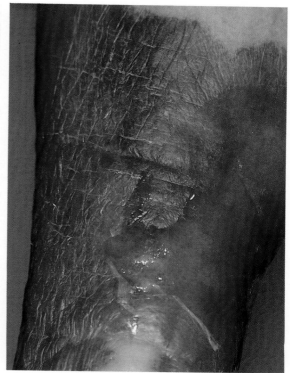

(b)

Fig. 10.10(a) & (b) Erysipelas and Cellulitis

Erysipelas is an acute, rapidly spreading inflammation of the superficial subcutaneous tissues and is due to haemolytic streptococci, usually Lancefield group A. It is commonest in adults and on the face, with hot, red, tender peau d'orange, and a distinct raised advancing edge, as seen in (a).

Cellulitis is a similar process caused by streptococci, staphylococci and occasionally other organisms such as *Bacteroides* and *Haemophilus influenzae* (the latter usually in a child). It is commonest in adults, often on a leg, and may spread extremely quickly to produce a large, hot, swollen tender area with lymphangitis, fever and malaise. The borders are less well defined than in erysipelas, probably because deeper subcutaneous tissues are involved. Epidermal necrosis often results in blistering, erosion and ulceration, and extensive deep necrosis can occur if treatment is delayed, as in (b). Much more rapid spread occurs if the infection spreads along fascial planes (necrotizing fasciitis).

Histologically, the dermis and subcutaneous fat are markedly oedematous and show dilatation of both blood and lymph vessels in the affected areas. A diffuse, often light, infiltration by neutrophil polymorphs is present throughout, but tending to concentrate around blood vessels. Streptococci are present in dermis, subcutaneous tissue and lymphatics.

Fig. 10.11. Folliculitis and boils

Folliculitis most commonly occurs in the beard area, on the thighs and buttocks, and is usually due to *Staphylococcus aureus*. The infection is confined to follicles and consists of multiple 1–2 mm diameter papules or pustules with a central hair. Larger lesions occur when the folliculitis is due to Gram-negative organisms (*E. coli*, *Klebsiella*). Boils also result from staphylococcal infection of hair follicles, but begin as often single deeper, larger, painful, red follicular nodules. The pustular centre becomes necrotic and the follicle is destroyed leaving a scar.

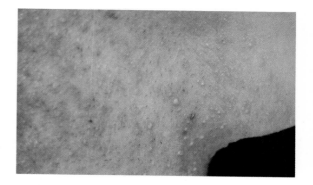

Fig. 10.12 Superficial folliculitis

Bacterial infection of the hair follicle may affect the upper portion of the follicle from sebaceous gland opening to surface, or the lower parts of the follicle from its base to the sebaceous gland opening. In the acute forms there is a perifollicular neutrophil infiltrate associated with abscess formation in the follicle. In superficial folliculitis, as here, the abscess occurs at the follicular opening, producing a small subcorneal pustule (arrow) through which the hair protrudes. In acute deep folliculitis the abscess is at the base of the follicle and often spreads out into adjacent subcutis ('furuncle' or boil). In the chronic forms of superficial and deep folliculitis, the abscess formation is persistent and produces more extensive necrosis. In addition to neutrophils, there are increasing numbers of lymphocytes and plasma cells in the infiltrate, and the abscess wall becomes lined by granulation tissue. Healing is by fibrosis leading to scarring and permanent loss of hair formation in affected follicles.

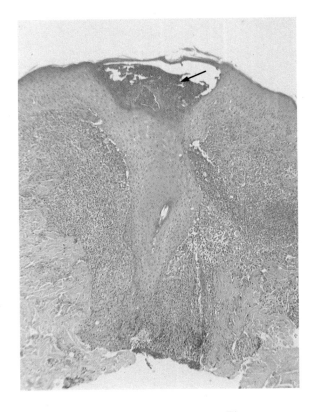

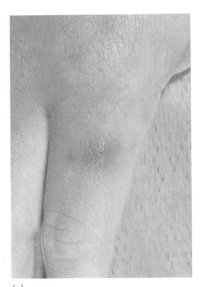

(a)

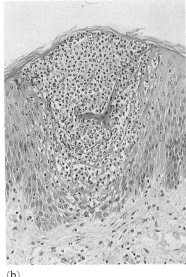

(b)

Fig. 10.13(a) & (b) Gonococcal and meningococcal skin lesions

In gonococcaemia there are usually small numbers (5–20) of vesicles or pustules, usually 1–5 mm in diameter, which are often haemorrhagic. They occur at the periphery and are most common on the fingers (a). Each vesicle or pustule has an erythematous base. The rash is usually associated with a flitting arthritis. The photographs show lesions from a case of chronic gonococcaemia.

In acute meningococcaemia, lesions are usually widespread, and are transiently macular or papular before becoming petechial; the characteristic clinical features are largely the result of widespread thrombosis in the small blood vessels in the skin, usually part of a generalized, disseminated intravascular coagulation. This is illustrated and discussed in more detail in Chapter 12. In chronic meningococcaemia lesions occur in crops with the fever and last for several days before remitting. They are usually macules or papules which are usually purpuric too, but larger tender nodules, petechiae or pustules may occur. In the skin lesion of chronic meningococcal (and gonococcal) bacteraemia, there is a neutrophilic vasculitis affecting small dermal blood vessels. Necrosis of vessel walls, extravasation of blood, and vascular occulusion by fibrin thrombi, may all occur but are much less frequent and less severe than in acute meningococcal lesions.

Mycobacterial infections in the skin

Because of their waxy capsule, mycobacteria are resistant to destruction by neutrophil enzymes, and the body mounts a predominantly histiocytic response to them, usually in the form of a chronic granulomatous reaction. Both conditions are discussed and illustrated in the chapter on granulomatous diseases in skin (see Ch. 11).

Spirochaetal infections of skin

Like the mycobacteria, spirochaetal organisms are resistant to destruction by neutrophils in the acute inflammatory reaction, and usually evoke a chronic inflammatory response in which histiocytes, lymphocytes and plasma cells are the predominant inflammatory cells. Depending on the nature of the organism, the stage of the infection, and the degree of resistance of the patient, there is a variable degree of immunological reaction to spirochaetal infection. This produces a very variable clinical and histological picture. The most frequently encountered Treponemal disease producing skin lesions is syphilis (due to *T. pallidum*); yaws (due to *T. pertenue*) and pinta (due to *T. carateum*) occur in tropical climes but are rare in temperate zones.

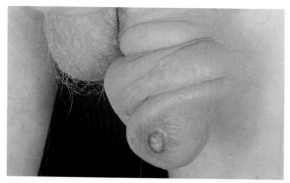

(a)

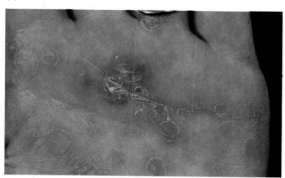

(b)

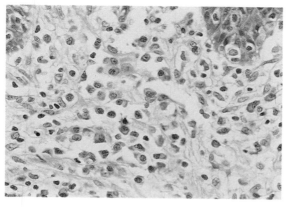

(c)

Fig. 10.14(a), (b) & (c) Syphilis

The primary lesion (chancre) is a painless nodule which develops into an ulcer with raised, indurated edges and little surrounding inflammation unless it is secondarily infected. It is located at the site of inoculation and so is usually found on the penis (a) or vulva. *Secondary skin lesions* usually develop 6–8 weeks later and the rash is often widespread and extremely variable; it may be macular, papular, pustular or papulosquamous, and often involves the palms (b) and soles. In adults it is never vesicular. Flattened moist papules in the flexures and on genitalia (condylomata lata) contain numerous spirochaetes and so are highly infective, as are lesions on mucous membranes. *Tertiary lesions* are usually nodular and ulcerated, and usually develop within 10 years or so of the initial infection.

The chancre shows a localized, dense collection of plasma cells and lymphocytes in the upper dermal blood vessels, most of which show severe endothelial swelling. At the edge of the lesion, the lymphoplasmacytic infiltrate is less dense and is mainly concentrated around blood vessels. At the peak of the nodule, the epidermis becomes spongiotic and thinned, and populated by inflammatory cells migrating upwards from upper dermis; central ulceration follows, although the epidermis remains intact (even acanthotic) at the periphery of the lesion. Following central ulceration, the histological appearances may be modified by secondary infection, trauma or ill-advised topical applications, but the cellular infiltrate remains predominantly plasma-celled.

In secondary syphilis skin lesions, the major histological feature is again a heavy plasma cell infiltrate in the upper dermis around prominent, thick-walled vessels showing endothelial swelling (c), but there are variable degrees of epidermal change depending on whether the lesion is macular, papular, or papulosquamous. Histologically, as well as clinically, secondary syphilis is a great mimic, and may show features resembling a wide range of inflammatory skin disorders such as psoriasis and lichen planus. In persistent nodular lesions, giant cell granulomata may be present.

FUNGAL INFECTIONS

The keratin layer forms a good barrier against fungal invasion, although fungi are commonly present on the skin surface as commensals. Fungi produce pathological changes in the skin in three main patterns: (i) superficial epidermal infection, (ii) infections of hair follicles and (iii) deep subcutaneous infections. Superficial infections with dermatophytes (Epidermophyton, Microsporum, Trichophyton) are common and clinical diagnosis straightforward, as is the case with infection due to Pityrosporum and Candida. Folliculitis due to fungi is less common but appears to be on the increase; immunosuppressed patients seem to be most prone. Deep fungal infections are much more serious but are uncommon in the UK, and consequently clinical diagnosis can be difficult.

Superficial dermatophytosis

Superficial fungal infections of the skin are extremely common, but the clinical presentation can be very varied. The most common are summarized in Table 10.3.

Table 10.3   Common superficial fungal infections of skin

Name	Fungus	Site	Appearance
Tinea capitis	Microsporum Trichophyton	Scalp	Hair loss and scaling; rarely inflammation (kerion)
Tinea corporis	Microsporum	Trunk	Ringworm—annular lesion with red, scaly edge
Tinea facei	Trichophyton rubrum	Face	Ringworm—annular lesion with red, scaly edge
Tinea cruris	Trichophyton Epidermophyton	Groin and thigh	Red, scaly edge pigmentation
Tinea pedis	Trichophyton Epidermophyton	Feet and toes	Athlete's foot—erythema, scaling
Tinea of hands and nails	Trichophyton rubrum	Hands and nails	Scaly, dry, peeling nail crumbling
Pityriasis versicolor	Pityrosporum orbiculare	Upper trunk	Hypo- and hyperpigmented macules. Fine scale.

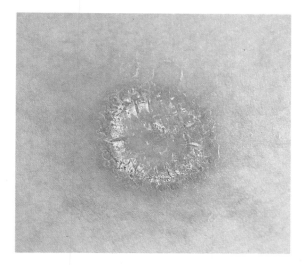

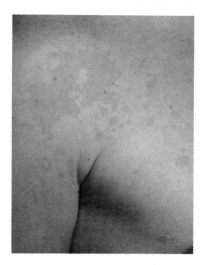

Fig. 10.15. Tinea corporis
This infection is mainly caused by *Microsporum canis* and *Trichophyton rubrum*. Annular lesions with raised red edge, occasionally papulovesicular, show characteristic central clearing with hypopigmentation.

Fig. 10.16. Pityriasis versicolor
This infection is due to *Pityrosporum orbiculare* which exists normally as a non-pathogenic rounded yeast, but develops elongated hyphal forms in pityriasis versicolor. It appears as irregular brown macules which enlarge to become confluent producing extensive patches. In patients with genetically dark or sun-tanned skin, the patches may be hypopigmented. It is largely confined to the upper trunk.

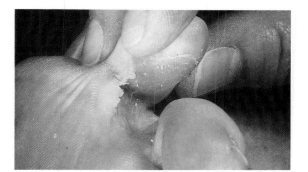

Fig. 10.17. Tinea pedis
There are two clinical patterns according to the causative organism. Infections by *Trichophyton mentagrophytes* produce fissuring and maceration between the toes, but on the rest of the foot the rash is itchy, erythematous and vesicular. Infections by *Trichophyton rubrum* produce redness and scaling of the sole of the foot, with painful fissuring between the toes. Nail involvement and destruction is most frequent with *T. rubrum* infections.

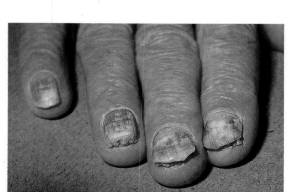

Fig. 10.18. Tinea of hands
Almost always due to *Trichophyton rubrum*, this is unilateral and presents as reddening of the palms with scaling and peeling of surface keratin. Co-existent nail involvement is common, and appears as whitish thickening and crumbling of the nail. Tinea of the hands and fingernails may co-exist with tinea of the feet and toe-nails.

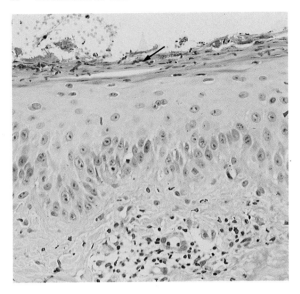

Fig. 10.19. Histology of the dermatophytoses
The histological diagnosis can be difficult on tissue sections,
particularly if a fungal lesion is not suspected clinically.
This is because the dermatophytic fungi do not stain clearly
with the routine H & E stain, and they can be easily missed
unless they are present in very large numbers or unless a
special stain (e.g. PAS, Grocott-Gomori methenamine
silver) is used. Better results can often be obtained by
examining scrapings of the surface scale, mounted in 30%
potassium hydroxide, under the microscope.

When present in a histological section, fungi are almost
always confined to the keratin layer, and rarely seem to
infiltrate the prickle cell layer, although they may be found
in hair follicles.

The tissue reaction to the presence of fungi is often
minimal, particularly at the centre of the patch; the most
active changes are seen at the expanding edge of the lesion,
particularly where it is red and raised. At this site there may
be a mild, non-specific upper dermal perivascular infiltrate
with lymphocytes and occasionally mild spongiosis. The
most dramatic histological changes are seen in the vesicular
lesions on the feet in tinea pedis due to *Trichophyton
mentagrophytes*; the epidermis contains numerous
spongiotic vesicles, and eosinophils may be numerous in the
epidermis and upper dermis in early itchy lesions;
secondary bacterial infection is not uncommon, and the
vesicles may become filled with neutrophils. The surprise
finding of eosinophils in the epidermis in an otherwise
non-specific dermatitis reaction should always stimulate the
pathologist to ask for special stains for fungi.

In the photomicrograph, note the fungal hyphae in the
keratin layer demonstrated by the PAS reaction (arrow).
There is no epidermal abnormality, and little associated
inflammation.

Fungal folliculitis

Fungal infection of the hair follicles may be due to infection by *Pityrosporum* or *Trichophyton rubrum*.
Folliculitis may also occur in some tinea corporis or tinea capitis lesions, usually where inflammation is severe,
e.g. in 'kerion'. *Pityrosporum folliculitis* usually occurs on the upper trunk, neck and arms in the form of small,
itchy, red papules or pustules. It is particularly common and extensive in immunosuppressed patients, and is
becoming a frequently observed skin lesion in patients with the acquired immune deficiency syndrome (AIDS).
Each affected follicle is distended with keratin in which large numbers of round, yeast-like organisms can be
seen; the wall of the follicle is usually infiltrated by mixed inflammatory cells, and there may be foreign body
giant cells in the infiltrate around the damaged follicle. *Trichophyton rubrum folliculitis* appears as a raised red
plaque with an irregular bumpy surface due to the enlarged inflamed follicles or as individual follicular papules;
it is most common on the lower leg and mainly occurs in women who also have tinea pedis due to *T. rubrum*.
Histologically, distended and inflamed follicles contain fungi, and there is a very florid perifollicular
inflammatory cell infiltrate in which fungi can be found, particularly in association with multinucleate giant
cells or small neutrophil aggregates.

Candida in skin

Candida infection of buccal mucosa is common, but involvement of the skin and nails is less frequent. Flexures,
perineal skin and corners of the mouth are the areas most commonly affected. The lesion appears as a moist, red
oedematous plaque with 2–3 mm satellite papules and pustules at its edges. The earliest lesion is an intra-
epidermal pustule, usually subcorneal, around which the epidermis may show spongiosis, and the underlying
dermis shows a florid mixed inflammatory infiltrate, mainly around dilated vessels. Again, the presence of
unexpected numbers of eosinophils, in both the dermis and the pustules, should arouse suspicion of a fungal
infection.

Deep fungal infections

These can occur in immunosuppressed patients, and histological diagnosis is often crucial. The clinical
appearance of deep mycotic lesions is extremely variable, from the swelling, induration and draining sinus
tracks of actinomycosis, nocardiosis and mycetoma (Madurella), to the erythematous pustules, papules, nodules
and plaques of cryptococcosis, and the mucosal ulcerations of the nasopharynx seen in histoplasmosis.

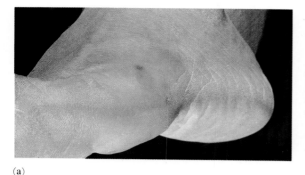

(a)

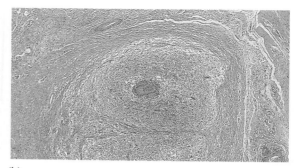

(b)

Fig. 10.20(a), (b) & (c). Madura foot

Clinically, this presents as extensive soft tissue swelling and induration of the foot, as in (a), and X-ray often shows evidence of bone destruction. Large deep abscess cavities constantly discharge onto the surface through sinuses.

The histological appearances are characteristic, providing the biopsy has been substantial and deep enough to include the abscesses in the deep dermis and subcutis. There is usually considerable fibrosis and chronic inflammation within which are found abscesses in the form of suppurating granulomas, that is, collections of neutrophil pus cells surrounded by a histiocytic granulomatous reaction (b) (see Ch. 11). Examination of the abscess cavities will reveal the causative organism in the form of characteristic colonies of either Actinomyces or Madurella (c), here stained prominently by the PAS method (arrow).

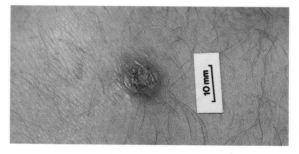

PROTOZOAL INFECTIONS

The only organisms to produce significant skin lesions belong to the Leishmania group, transmitted by sandflies.

Fig. 10.21(a) & (b). Cutaneous leishmaniasis ('oriental sore')

The commonest form seen in the UK is acute cutaneous leishmaniasis due to *L. tropica*, and has usually been acquired in the Mediterranean, Middle or Far East, or Central or Southern America. The lesion is usually a single, 5–10 mm diameter papule at the site of the bite of the sandfly, and enlarges over 1–2 months into a dark red-brown oedematous and often ulcerated nodule (a). The disease may become chronic in the elderly, but usually heals within 18 months with scarring. New lesions occasionally occur around old healed ones, when the appearance can resemble lupus vulgaris (*Leishmania recidivans*) and there may be multiple lesions when immunity is poor (disseminated cutaneous leishmaniasis). Lesions due to *L. Brasiliensis* are initially like those of *L. tropica* but are much more likely to involve mouth and nasopharynx (American mucocutaneous leishmaniasis). Direct skin involvement in visceral leishmaniasis (due to *L. Donovani*) occurs in partially treated and chronic disease with depigmented macules and subsequently nodules.

There is a dense infiltration of the dermis by macrophages and some lymphocytes and plasma cells. In early lesions the macrophages may contain large numbers of *Leishmania tropica* organisms which can usually be easily seen as small dark dots within the cytoplasm in an H & E-stained section. They are also well demonstrated by the Giemsa stain. However, it is important to realise that this classical appearance is only seen in the early stages of the lesion. Once the nodule ulcerates, secondary changes blur the picture and the infected macrophages become less numerous, the inflammatory infiltrate becoming dominated

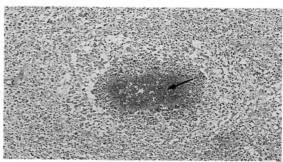

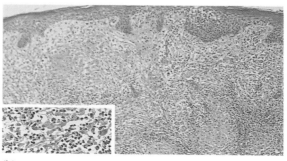

(b)

by neutrophils, lymphocytes and plasma cells. Sometimes a histiocytic dermal granulomatous reaction occurs in chronic cutaneous leishmaniasis (b) but there is much less necrosis and organisms are rare (see inset).

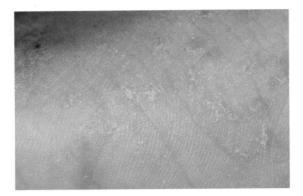

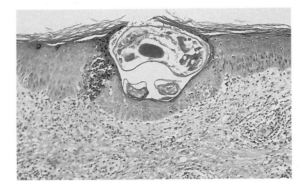

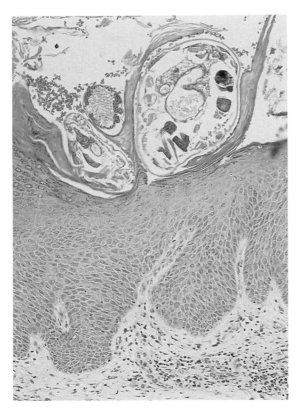

PARASITIC INFESTATIONS

Fig. 10.22(a), (b) & (c). Scabies

This is caused by the mite *Sarcoptes scabiei*; the female burrows into the stratum corneum, leaving visible tracks especially on the palms, wrists and fingers (a). In addition, an itchy widespread papular rash can occur; these papules may develop into nodules and often persist for weeks after successful treatment.

Histologically, most biopsies of scabies burrows are devoid of mites unless the end of the burrow is sectioned. The burrow through which the mite has already passed is intra- or subcorneal in location, but the terminal vesicle occupied by the mite involves the full thickness of the epidermis. The epidermis around the mite shows variable spongiosis and a usually scanty infiltration with inflammatory cells in which eosinophils may be prominent; a similar infiltrate may be present in the associated upper dermis. Occasionally, in severe reactions, there may be small eosinophilic aggregates within the epidermis close to the burrow. Inflammatory cell infiltration is less marked in the region of 'old' burrow through which the mite passed some time previously, and is mainly lymphocytic, although occasional persisting eosinophils and mast cells may be seen.

The itchy papular lesions may not contain mites, but show a non-specific upper dermal chronic inflammatory cell infiltrate in which eosinophils and mast cells may be numerous. In some larger nodules and papules there may be large numbers of atypical histiocytes and lymphocytes, mimicking lymphoma. However, these lesions usually show vascular changes such as endothelial cell swelling and proliferation, and vessel wall thickening, suggesting a chronic inflammatory or allergic basis. Some of the largest, long-standing nodules may be histologically indistinguishable from lymphomatoid papulosis (see Fig. 22.8).

In extensive or 'Norwegian' scabies, vast numbers of mites are seen in the stratum corneum (c). The underlying epidermis shows marked acanthosis and there is a heavy dermal chronic inflammatory cell infiltrate.

11. Granulomatous lesions in the skin

Introduction

Dermatologists and histopathologists mean different things when they use the term 'granulomatous'. Clinicians use the word to describe chronic, red-brown, firm, raised lesions, either nodules, papules or plaques, which blanch on pressure to reveal paler brown lesions. Histopathologists use the word to describe a particular pattern of chronic inflammation in which the predominant inflammatory cell is the macrophage (histiocyte), with variable numbers of lymphocytes. In such histiocytic chronic inflammatory reactions, occasionally the histiocytes aggregate to form a discrete circumscribed mass (a granuloma), in which some histiocytes fuse together to form large, multinucleate giant cells. When giant cell formation is prominent, the reaction is called a giant cell granulomatous reaction.

Pathological basis of giant cell granulomatous reactions.

Granulomatous inflammatory reactions are usually seen in circumstances in which the more usual acute inflammatory (neutrophilic) reaction is incapable of dealing satisfactorily with the damaging agent. The main cause of this is the inability of neutrophils to either phagocytose the agent, or, having phagocytosed it, is unable to destroy it with its lysosomal enzymes. Histiocytes/macrophages are much longer-lived than neutrophils and are more tenacious phagocytosers; thus a histiocytic granulomatous inflammatory reaction represents a second line of defence and is invoked quickly after an initial acute inflammatory reaction fails to eradicate or neutralize a damaging agent. The most likely damaging agents to resist and survive neutrophil phagocytosis and lysosomal enzyme destruction are:

1. **Bacteria** which have a protective coat capable of withstanding neutrophil enzymes during the short life-span of the white cell. The most important group of organisms is the Mycobacteria, which have a thick, lipid external capsule. Thus, diseases such as tuberculosis and leprosy are characterized by a chronic inflammatory granulomatous reaction in the skin; see Figures 11.1, 11.2). The particular pattern of the reaction, e.g. the severity of tissue necrosis, the number and nature of the histiocytes present, the degree of lymphocyte infiltration, is dependent on a number of factors, the most important of which are the nature of the damaging agent, its duration, and the immunological status of the patient.

2. **Fungi** which are partly resistant to neutrophil destruction. Superficial fungal infections of skin rarely excite a florid reaction, but deep fungal dermatoses often show a histiocytic reaction, sometimes in the form of a 'suppurating granuloma', in which a collection of neutrophils is surrounded by a histiocytic granulomatous reaction.

3. **Exogenous foreign material**, either organic or inorganic. Inert inorganic material is usually introduced into the skin accidentally by trauma, e.g. beryllium granulomas in metal workers. Other materials in this category which can excite a granulomatous reaction include other metal particles, metallic compounds used as tattoo pigments, and non-metallic elements such as silica (in the skin, particularly in the form of glass splinters; elsewhere in the body, talc and silicaceous dusts are most important). In the skin, the most frequent non-infective organic material to produce this type of reaction is wood, usually in the form of a splinter or a thorn. Chitinous material, such as mouthparts from insects, often produces a very florid chronic inflammatory reaction with a mixed cellular infiltrate, including eosinophils; only in the very late stages is there a granulomatous type of reaction, and then fairly insignificant.

4. **Endogenous altered material**, usually degenerate collagen. This is the basis of granulomatous skin lesions such as rheumatoid nodules, granuloma annulare, and necrobiosis lipoidica. Less commonly, released lipid or keratin, and precipitated urate crystals can excite a granulomatous reaction. A histiocytic response is a variable late feature of some patterns of large-vessel vasculitis, and is particularly obvious in the variant known as 'giant cell', 'temporal' or 'cranial' arteritis in which the histiocytic giant cells appear to form in close proximity to disrupted and degenerate arterial elastic lamina.

5. **Unknown cause**, e.g. sarcoid.

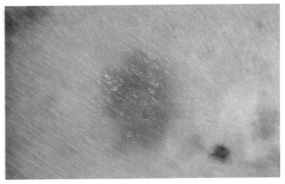

(a)

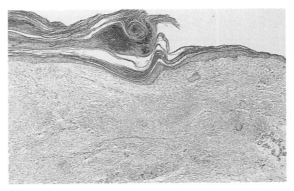

(b)

Fig. 11.1(a) & (b) Tuberculosis (Lupus vulgaris)

Lupus vulgaris is becoming increasingly rare. Most patients are elderly, and the lesions have usually been present for many years and may even be referred to by the patient as a birthmark. They consist of grouped, brownish papules or plaques, often with considerable previous destruction of adjacent skin and appendages, resulting in atrophy, and are commonest on face and proximal limbs.

Granulomata composed of histiocytes and giant cells, including Langhans types, are present in all layers of the dermis. They are mostly in the upper dermis, but may extend down into the upper subcutis. Caseation may be present but it is not invariable; the expanding granulomata may become semi-confluent and lead to destruction of skin appendages. There is usually a lymphocytic infiltrate around the granulomata, and long-standing lesions may show considerable irregular fibrosis, particularly when there has been ulceration of the overlying epidermis, and these secondary changes may obscure the granulomatous nature of the inflammation. Tubercle bacilli can rarely be identified in paraffin sections, and it is vital for the dermatologist to send half of the biopsy for culture. It is worth trying the fluorescent auramine-rhodamine method to detect acid-fast bacilli in a paraffin section, it offers a greater chance of success than the Ziehl-Neelsen method.

Fig. 11.2(a)–(f) Leprosy (*illustrations opposite*)

Leprosy is an extremely polymorphous disease and the physical signs in the skin vary with the intensity of the host response. In *tuberculoid leprosy*, when cell-mediated immunity is considerable, lesions are usually even, purple plaques with raised edges and an anaesthetic, depressed centre, or hypopigmented macules (a). Sweating is reduced or absent, and hair is usually lost because of follicular destruction. Infiltration of the skin of the face produces 'leonine' facies, and mucosal involvement, especially in the nose, can be severe. In *lepromatous leprosy*, macules are more numerous and ill-defined; there may be papules, nodules (b), and plaques too, are usually widespread, especially on limbs. These are not anaesthetic, but ulceration of lesions may result from peripheral neuropathy in progressive disease. A range of skin lesions between these two extremes occur in *borderline leprosy*.

In tuberculoid leprosy, histiocytic granulomata are found in all layers of the dermis (arrow in (c)) but are particularly found in the region of cutaneous nerves, hence the anaesthesia. Giant cells may be present, and there may be focal necrosis in some granulomata, particularly those associated with nerves (arrow in (d)). *M. leprae* can rarely be detected histologically in the skin in tuberculoid leprosy, so there is no certain way of distinguishing it from lupus vulgaris or sarcoid.

In lepromatous leprosy, there is an extensive infiltration of the mid-and lower dermis and upper subcutis by a mixture of large pale-staining, foamy histiocytic cells (lepra cells – arrows) and lymphocytes (e). *Mycobacterium leprae* can be found in large numbers within the lepra cells and in the large nerves, using the Wade-Fite stain (arrows in (f)). Skin appendages are destroyed, but nerves in the skin are well preserved.

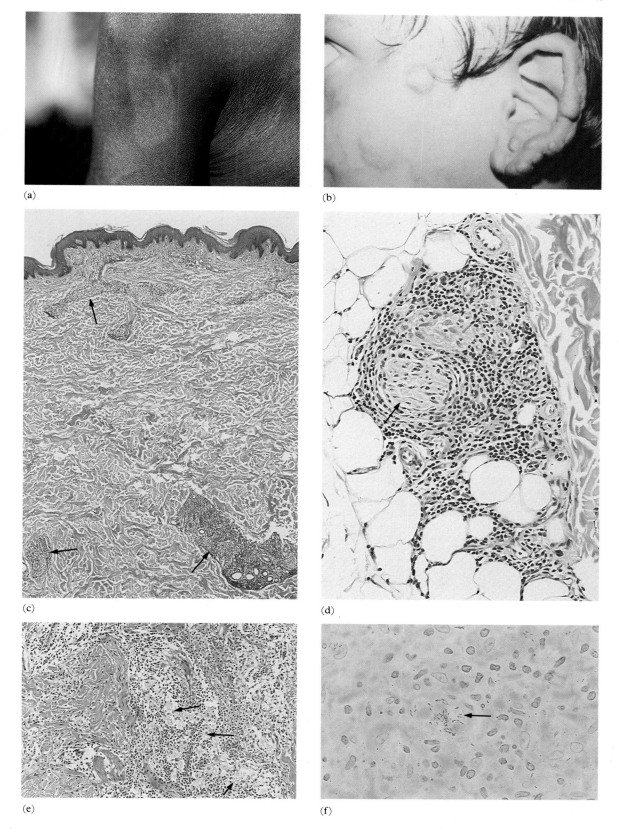

(a)

(b)

(c)

(d)

(e)

(f)

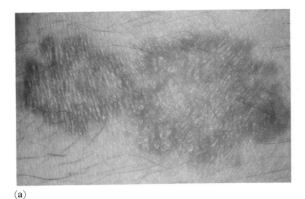

(a)

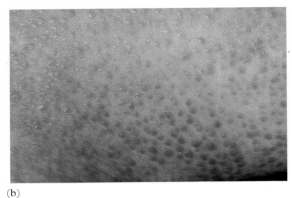

(b)

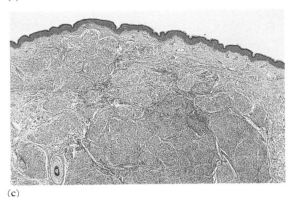

(c)

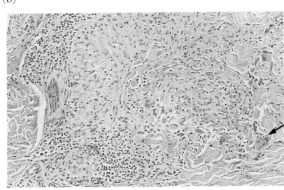

(d)

Fig. 11.3(a)–(d) Sarcoidosis

There are several distinct appearances to cutaneous sarcoidosis. Lupus pernio is persistent, purple, rubbery plaques and nodules on the tips of the nose, fingers and ears: it is strongly associated with chronic and severe nasal mucosal lesions, and with lung, eye and bone involvement. Fixed plaques with brown papules and nodules, and central atrophy, can occur, usually on trunk and limbs (a). Follicular granulomatous papules with hair loss (b), and inflammation in previous scars which become purple and swollen are less common. Although commonly associated with sarcoidosis, erythema nodosum is distinct and does not show sarcoid granuloma formation histologically. Despite this variety, the histological appearance is remarkably uniform and is characterized by the presence of florid histiocytic granulomata in the dermis and occasionally in subcutis. The granulomata are usually clearly defined but have a tendency to become confluent (c). Lymphocytes form a variable cuff around the cellular histiocytic granulomata; giant cells may be sparse (arrow in (d)), and there may be focal eosinophilic necrosis (not caseous) within some granulomata. In older lesions the granulomata are less florid and well-defined, and may be associated with fibrosis; large giant cells containing calcified Schauman bodies or asteroid bodies are particularly a feature of long-standing skin sarcoid lesions.

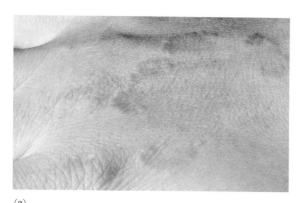

(a)

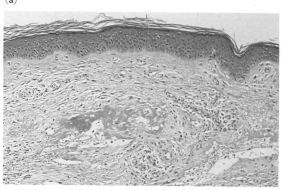

(b)

Fig. 11.4(a) & (b) Granuloma annulare

Lesions are most commonly found on the dorsum of the hands and feet in children and adolescents, but can occur at any site in the skin and at any age. They usually consist of flesh-coloured nodules, arranged in arcs and rings (a); as they expand they leave a purplish centre, and lesions resolve spontaneously. Occasionally there are solitary lesions, sometimes with a punctum rather like molluscum contagiosum, or diffuse flesh-coloured dermal nodules. Epidermal changes such as scaling are not a feature, but occasionally necrotic material (presumably damaged collagen) is extruded, so-called 'perforating granuloma annulare'. Histologically, there are small foci of degeneration of dermal collagen scattered throughout the mid- and lower dermis (b). The degeneration is manifest as a change in the staining characteristics of the collagen with eosin, sometimes an intensification, sometimes a diminution; the fibres often appear swollen. Between the abnormal fibres there is a variable infiltrate of lymphocytes and histiocytes, and plump, spindle-shaped active fibroblasts are often prominent; histiocytes, lymphocytes and occasional giant cells usually surround these degenerate nodules, particularly the larger ones.

Less commonly, the lesions are fewer and larger; in these lesions the collagen is more degenerate and amorphous, and are surrounded by a prominent histiocytic and lymphocytic reaction in which giant cells may be numerous.

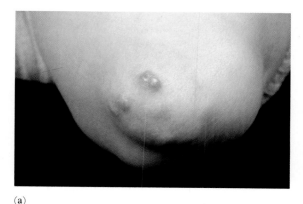

(a)

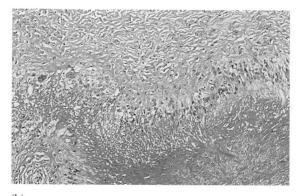

(b)

Fig. 11.5(a) & (b) Rheumatoid nodule

These are usually found over bony prominences (especially elbows) in patients with severe seropositive rheumatoid arthritis. They are rubbery, mobile nodules which may be subcutaneous or within the skin (a). Histologically, the nodules are composed of irregular areas of degenerate, highly eosinophilic material, mainly collagen, with a surrounding chronic inflammatory cell infiltrate in which large histiocytes often form a distinct, palisaded layer in contact with the degenerate collagen. Giant cells may be present but are rarely numerous (b).

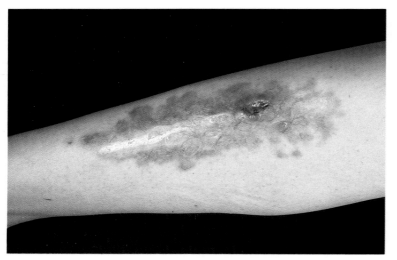

(a)

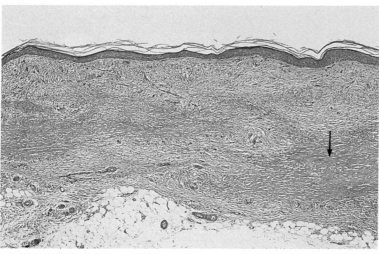

(b)

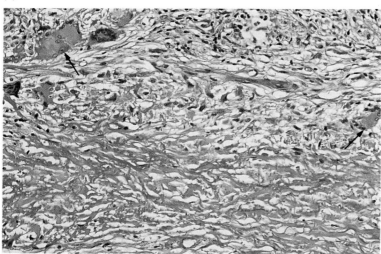

(c)

Fig. 11.6(a), (b) & (c) Necrobiosis lipoidica

The clinical appearance is usually striking, with yellowish, shiny, atrophic, depressed, telangiectatic plaques on the shins, which may ulcerate (a). Rarely, lesions occur at other sites, e.g. upper limbs and face. They evolve from much less striking brownish papules which slowly enlarge. There may be a raised translucent edge but the appearance is distinct from granuloma annulare, although they share many histological features. The relative risk of associated diabetes is negligible in granuloma annulare but considerable in necrobiosis, although most diabetics do not develop cutaneous necrobiosis lesions.

These lesions, like granuloma annulare, show areas of degeneration of collagen (necrobiosis) throughout the dermis, but with a tendency to be in the deeper levels of the dermis (arrow in (b)). They are surrounded and variably infiltrated by an inflammatory cell population in which lymphocytes and histiocytes predominate; giant cells are present (arrow) and may be numerous (c), particularly when the inflammatory cells are aggregated into granulomatous foci (granulomatous pattern of necrobiosis lipoidica). Because the areas of collagen degeneration are frequently located in the deep dermis, the inflammatory reaction often spills into the adipose tissue of the subcutis. Incorporation of lipid droplets into the foci of degeneration and inflammatory reaction results, and is claimed to be a useful distinguishing feature from granuloma annulare. In some variants, particularly those with a florid granulomatous reaction, the areas of collagen degeneration may be small, scanty and difficult to find.

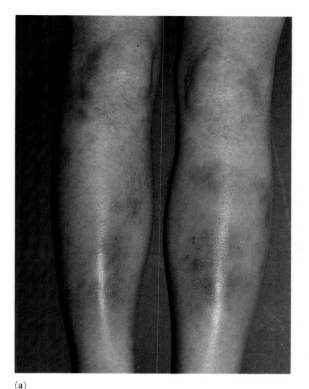

(a)

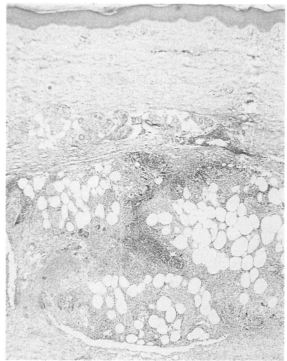

(b)

Fig. 11.7(a) (b) & (c) Erythema nodosum

Lesions develop acutely as extremely tender, elevated, hot red subcutaneous lumps, usually 2–5 cm across, on the shins (a), thighs, and occasionally arms. They last several weeks, leaving a bruise, as a result of vessel damage, and are usually accompanied by fever, arthralgia, and malaise. Common causes are sarcoidosis, or an immune reaction to a recent streptococcal infection. Drugs (sulphonamides especially), inflammatory bowel disease and other infectious causes (e.g. TB) occur, but are less common. The clinical appearances are so typical that the lesions are rarely biopsied.

The histological changes are those of an ill-defined inflammatory cell infiltrate, mainly of lymphocytes and histiocytes, in the subcutaneous fat. The most dense concentration of cells is in the connective tissue septa in upper subcutis, particularly around septal blood vessels (b). In early lesions, neutrophils may be present in large numbers, but the neutrophilic phase is transient. In nearly all lesions, a medium-sized vein showing heavy inflammation of its wall will be found, even though a number of levels of the biopsy may need to be examined. Giant cells (arrows) are usually present in the inflammatory infiltrate (c), particularly in long-standing lesions where the inflammation may be obviously granulomatous and the vessel inflammation less active.

A number of lesions can resemble erythema nodosum clinically and, in part, histologically as well. For reasons which are not entirely justified, these are often grouped together as 'nodular vasculitis', presumably because the lesions are clinically nodular and histologically have evidence of an active vasculitis. However, vessel inflammation is a frequent finding only in the clinically distinct lesions of erythema induratum, erythema nodosum, polyarteritis nodosa and superficial thrombophlebitis. The

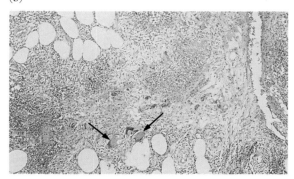

(c)

term 'nodular vasculitis' should be discouraged as a blanket term. *Erythema induratum* begins as bluish nodules on the calves, especially in middle-aged women, and the lesions usually ulcerate: they are very persistent. Histologically, there is an ill-defined focus of chronic granulomatous inflammation in the subcutaneous fat. The inflammatory cell infiltrate consists of histiocytes, lymphocytes and multinucleate giant cells. These are sometimes arranged into ill-defined nodular granulomata, but mainly insinuate into septa between subcutaneous adipose tissue where they are associated with fat necrosis and severe inflammatory damage to blood vessels, both arterial and venous. The vessels are thick-walled as a result of infiltration by inflammatory cells (mainly lymphocytes), and endothelial swelling leads to reduction of the lumen, a process sometimes complicated by thrombosis. When this occurs, areas of amorphous necrosis develop which may involve the overlying dermis leading to the ulceration observed clinically.

Miscellaneous granulomatous reactions in skin

Foreign body granulomas

The skin is frequently breached by minor acts of trauma, and exogenous foreign material introduced into dermis and subcutis; if the material is incapable of destruction by neutrophil polymorphs, as is usually the case, a giant cell granulomatous reaction frequently surrounds the foreign material. This is known as the foreign body giant cell reaction, and an example is illustrated in Fig 4.11. A common cause of foreign body granulomatous reaction to endogenous foreign material is seen around traumatized epidermal cysts where keratin has leaked into surrounding tissue following rupture of the cyst wall ('infected sebaceous cyst'). Urate crystals precipitated in the tissues in hyperuricaemic conditions such as gout also precipitate a foreign body giant cell reaction.

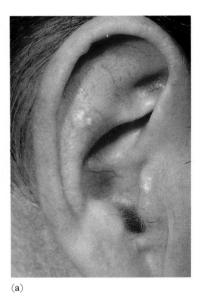

(a)

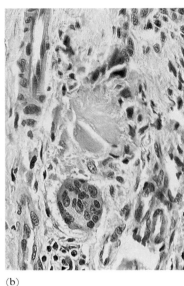

(b)

Fig. 11.8(a) & (b) Gout
Deposition of urate crystals in the subcutaneous tissue is frequent in untreated chronic gout and secondary hyperuricaemia. The deposits form a firm, raised, yellowish nodule, often with a narrow erythematous rim; small at the outset, they can become very large and ulcerate, discharging yellowish-white chalky or pasty material. They are most frequent on the fingers and toes, the elbow and the helix of the ear (a).

Histologically, there is a florid granulomatous giant cell reaction in subcutis and dermis, at the centre of which is amorphous pink material in which fine linear crystals of urate can be seen, providing they have not dissolved out during tissue processing. They are highly water-soluble and fixation in alcohol, followed by dehydration in changes of absolute alcohol, is advisable for any specimen in which gout is suspected. The crystals are refractile when viewed by polarizing microscopy.

Granulomatous reactions on the face

The histological finding of a giant cell granulomatous reaction is frequent in association with a wide range of lesions occurring on the face. It may be a result of trauma (e.g. squeezing, shaving) to common lesions such as comedones, small epidermal cysts, chronic folliculitis. Fragments of extruded hair shaft or keratin can sometimes be seen lying free in the dermis at the heart of the granulomatous reaction. Note that the condition known as *granuloma faciale* is not histologically granulomatous but shows features of vasculitis (see Fig. 12.4).

Two specific patterns of granulomatous lesion on the face are worthy of mention, granulomatous rosacea and lupus miliaris disseminata faciei.

Granulomatous rosacea is the name given to the papular pattern of rosacea when the papules are the result of a granulomatous inflammatory reaction around damaged hair follicles; Demodex fragments can often be found within the granulomatous area.

Lupus miliaris disseminata faciei (acne agminata) most commonly presents as small, red-brown papules in the eyelids and around the eyes, but may be more extensive and involve the cheeks, chin and forehead. The papules are persistent and usually heal after months or years with scarring. The histological appearances are dramatic, with a round area of central caseation surrounded by a florid giant cell granulomatous reaction (see Fig. 4.4). The lesions are well-circumscribed and are located in the upper dermis. Despite their name and their resemblance to classical caseating tuberculosis (they are more tubercle-like than the lesions in lupus vulgaris), they are unrelated to tuberculosis.

12. Vasculitic skin disorders

Introduction

It is important to define precisely what is meant when the term *vasculitis* is used; it implies an inflammatory destruction of the walls of blood vessels, which will leave the vessel wall damaged and often non-functional after the acute episode is over. It is important to distinguish it histologically from the blood vessel changes seen in non-specific acute and chronic inflammation. In *acute inflammation* blood vessels play a vital part in the pathophysiological mechanisms involved in the formation of the acute inflammatory exudate. In the early stages of the process, small blood vessels (mainly capillaries) become persistently dilated, and alterations in the pattern of blood flow within them occur. At the same time the vessel wall shows swelling and separation of the normally thin flat endothelial cells, and the vessel basement membrane becomes more permeable. Plasma water and proteins pass through the vessel wall from the lumen to the extra-vascular tissues, and circulating neutrophils concentrate and stick on the endothelial cells ("margination") before passing through the vessel walls to the exterior. One of the soluble plasma proteins, fibrinogen, polymerises into insoluble long fibrils of fibrin once it has passed outside the vessel wall. In this way, the acute inflammatory exudate (water, proteins, insoluble fibrin and neutrophils) is formed outside the vessels in the area of tissue damage. With persistence of the damaging stimulus, the nature of the exudate changes, fibrin and neutrophils becoming replaced by reparative granulation and fibrous tissue and lymphocytes, with some macrophages and plasma cells; these are characteristic of a *chronic inflammatory response*. In some inflammations with an allergic basis, eosinophils may be numerous.

Thus histological examination of inflamed skin will invariably show evidence of an inflammatory process, with either acute inflammatory cells (i.e. neutrophils), or chronic inflammatory cells (i.e. lymphocytes, macrophages and plasma cells) around dermal blood vessels. Many photomicrographs in this atlas show such perivascular accumulations of inflammatory cells, but this is not true vasculitis.

Histological evidence of true vasculitis

In the pathophysiological changes of acute inflammation outlined above, the vessels usually regain their normal structure and function, whereas in true vasculitis the vessel walls are damaged. Histological evidence that the vessel is likely to be permanently damaged is based on two findings:
1. Visible evidence of necrosis of the components of the vessel wall.
2. Inflammatory cells within the components of the vessel wall.

Necrosis of vessel wall

In acute vasculitis, the most common visible manifestation of vessel wall necrosis is the change known as *fibrinoid necrosis* (see Figs. 4.10, 12.1, 12.2), in which the normal structures of the wall (endothelial cells, basement membrane and smooth muscle cells) cannot be seen. Instead, the wall is replaced by a deeply eosinophilic, amorphous material called *fibrinoid* because it shows many of the staining characteristics of fibrin. It is probably a mixture of fibrin, fibrinogen and mixed plasma proteins including complement, trapped in the damaged vessel wall; it suggests that the affected vessel is damaged beyond normal repair, particularly when the vessel is small (e.g. capillary or arteriole) and the damage is circumferential. In larger vessels, such as elastic arteries, the necrosis may only affect one segment of the vessel's circumference and there may be potential for recovery of the vessel as a functional unit, although the affected segment remains permanently scarred. Such old, scarred lesions can be demonstrated most clearly by the use of a connective tissue stain such as the Elastic-van Gieson which demonstrates disruption of the elastic lamina and replacement of the smooth muscle cells by collagenous scar tissue.

Inflammatory cells in vessel wall

Further evidence of true vasculitis is the presence of inflammatory cells within, and expanding the wall of, a vessel. Margination of neutrophils to the endothelial lining, and perivascular accumulations of inflammatory cells, do *not* constitute evidence of wall invasion and are not indicative of a vasculitis. A useful guide to the likely nature and cause of a vasculitis is afforded by the type of inflammatory cell which is infiltrating the wall. In this chapter, vasculitis will be discussed under the headings *neutrophilic vasculitis, lymphocytic vasculitis* and *histiocytic/giant cell vasculitis*. This division is not precise since most vessel wall inflammations contain a mixture of inflammatory cells and the lesion is classified according to the predominant cell present. Furthermore, the nature of the cell present may depend on the age of the vasculitic lesion at the time of biopsy; for example, the most common type of histiocytic and giant cell vasculitis is temporal (or giant cell) arteritis (see Fig. 12.8) in which there is always a neutrophil and eosinophil component. In early lesions, neutrophils and eosinophils predominate, and mononuclear or multinucleate histiocytes are scanty.

NEUTROPHILIC VASCULITIS

When dermatologists describe a skin lesion as vasculitic, they are usually describing the physical signs resulting from neutrophilic vasculitis affecting the small vessels of the upper dermis. Involvement of larger deep dermal and subcutaneous vessels is much less common. Neutrophilic vasculitis confined to large veins is rare, and is usually confined to early lesions. In later lesions, lymphocytes and histiocytes become admixed.

Causes of neutrophilic vasculitis

The causes of neutrophilic vasculitis affecting medium and large arteries are few, and polyarteritis nodosa or one of its variants is much the most common. Neutrophilic vasculitis of small blood vessels, such as capillaries and venules, is common and has a large number of causes; however, the histological features are virtually identical, whatever the cause. Vascular damage probably results from deposition within the walls of antigen-antibody complexes; immunoglobulins, complement components and fibrinogen can be demonstrated in the vessel walls in early active lesions in most cases.

A number of clearly defined small-vessel vasculitis syndromes exists, including Henoch-Schönlein purpura, hypocomplementaemic vasculitis with or without cryoglobulinaemia, and rheumatoid and SLE vasculitis; small vessel vasculitis may also be due to drugs or septicaemias. Systemic involvement is quite common: joints, muscles, central nervous system, kidney, and gastrointestinal tract may all be involved.

Small vessel neutrophilic vasculitis

The characteristic lesion is *palpable purpura*, a haemorrhagic urticated papule, which may become necrotic and blister (see Fig. 12.1), usually on the limbs. There may be a range of lesions present, from urticaria to erythematous nodules, especially in less acute forms of the disease. The vasculitic changes are usually confined to small capillaries and venules in the upper and mid-dermis. The vessel walls show extensive or patchy fibrinoid necrosis of their walls, associated with infiltration of the walls by live and dead neutrophils, which are also present as a cuff around the vessel. The ratio of live to dead neutrophils varies, but the nuclear remnants of dead neutrophils can almost always be found and are often numerous. They take the form of minute, haematoxyphilic scattered fragments, sometimes called 'nuclear dust'. This pattern of nuclear breakdown after cell death is widely seen throughout the body and, in all other circumstances, is termed karyorrhexis, but in dermatopathology has acquired the inaccurate name leukocytoclasis. Neutrophilic vasculitis has thus been termed leukocytoclastic vasculitis, a phrase which is probably superfluous. Small vessels showing active neutrophilic vasculitis usually show perivascular oedema, and red cells are often extravasated producing the purpuric lesions seen clinically. In some cases of small vessel neutrophilic vasculitis, eosinophils may be mixed with the neutrophil population, particularly when the vasculitis has an allergic cause (e.g. drug reaction).

Fig. 12.1(a), (b) & (c) Small vessel neutrophilic vasculitis (*illustrations opposite*)
This example is from a patient with Henoch-Schönlein purpura. Clinically, the lesions appear as erythematous and purpuric papules, usually 2–3 mm in diameter, mainly on the extremities and buttocks. It is common in children and adolescents, but occurs at all ages. The photomicrographs show that the vasculitis is confined to the small vessels in the upper and mid-dermis. The high power photomicrograph is of a vessel showing focal fibrinoid necrosis, heavy neutrophilic infiltration of the vessel wall and haemotoxyphilic fragments of nuclear debris from dead neutrophils (karyorrhexic nuclear dust). Note the oedema around the vessel, and the extravasated red cells.

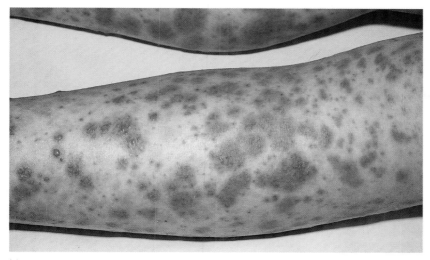

(a)

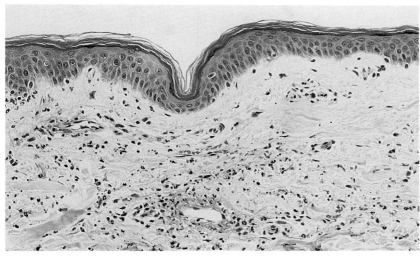

(b)

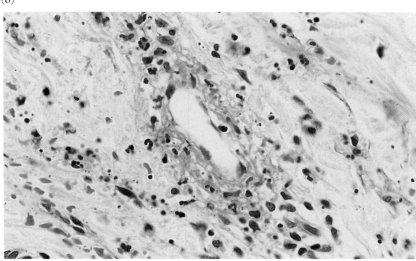

(c)

Large vessel neutrophilic vasculitis

The main vessels to be involved are the medium-sized arteries in the dermis and subcutis, but there may also be an associated small vessel vasculitis in nearby upper dermis, depending on the cause. Clinically, the characteristic lesions are tender nodules, sometimes subcutaneous, in association with livedo reticularis. Nodules form at the site of vasculitis and may follow the course of the vessel involved; occlusion of the affected vessel by inflammation or thrombosis produces ischaemia which may lead to skin necrosis and ulceration. Livedo is local cyanosis due to decreased flow in superficial vessels and so is most noticeable at the watershed between areas of supply where flow is slowest. Livedo occurs frequently in association with connective tissue disorders, especially lupus erythematosus, dermatomyositis and cutaneous polyarteritis. The inflammatory cell infiltrate originating in the vessel wall may spread extensively in the surrounding dermis and subcutaneous fat, producing a raised nodule. Some types of large vessel arteritis, particularly polyarteritis nodosa, have a large number of eosinophils in the infiltrate. Thus in the early stages, the vessel wall shows a mixed infiltrate of neutrophils and eosinophils throughout all layers splitting the muscle fibres, associated with varying degrees of fibrinoid necrosis. Perivascular oedema is less marked than in small vessel vasculitis, but the perivascular cellular infiltrate is usually more prominent. Nuclear debris from dead neutrophils is again present, but is less apparent than in small vessel vasculitis, being overwhelmed by the large number of viable neutrophils and eosinophils present when a large vessel is involved. At a later stage, the inflammatory cell population in the wall may become less prominently neutrophilic and eosinophilic, and increasing numbers of lymphocytes and histiocytes appear. Histiocytic giant cells are particularly prominent when the artery is one with an internal elastic lamina, being closely associated with the necrotic fragments of elastin (see section on histiocytic/giant cell vasculitis below).

(a)

Fig. 12.2(a)–(d) Large vessel neutrophilic vasculitis
((b) – (d) opposite)
The illustrated example is from a case of polyarteritis nodosa; note the reddish ill-defined nodules and the hint of livedo (arrow in (a)). Photomicrographs (b) and (c) show the distribution of the necrotizing vasculitis with a prominent vessel in mid-dermis showing extensive fibrinoid necrosis (arrows). There is also acute neutrophilic vasculitis in some upper dermal vessels. Photomicrograph (d) shows a larger artery from the subcutis of the same patient. Note the extensive destruction of the artery wall by a combination of fibrinoid necrosis and heavy neutrophil infiltrate. The lumen is occluded.

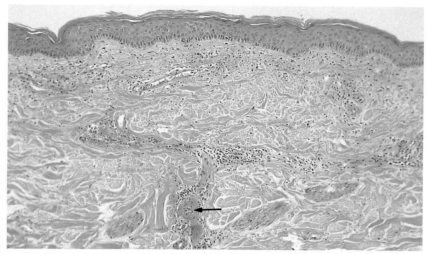

(b)

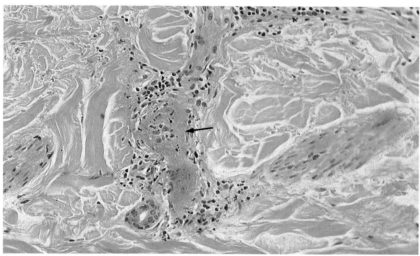

(c)

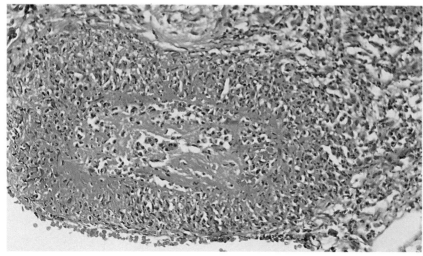

(d)

Conditions with a secondary neutrophilic vasculitis

Histological vasculitis may be found in association with a number of conditions in which it is obviously secondary to some other lesion. For example, neutrophilic vasculitis can be seen in the upper dermis beneath viral epidermal blisters such as varicella and herpes zoster and beneath traumatic epidermal ulcers in dermatitis artefacta. It can also rarely be seen in lesions such as granuloma annulare and necrobiosis lipoidica. However, there are a few conditions in which a neutrophilic vasculitis is seen where it may be the primary lesion, although the pathogenesis is uncertain. Examples include pyoderma gangrenosum, granuloma faciale and erythema elevatum diutinum; the latter two conditions do not have systemic involvement.

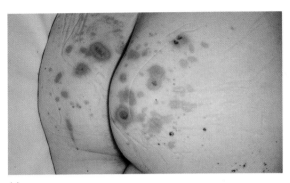

(a)

Fig. 12.3(a), (b) & (c) Pyoderma gangrenosum

This usually begins as a tender, red, enlarging nodule, the centre of which becomes necrotic, forming an ulcer with a sloughing base (arrow in (a)). Characteristically, the edge of the ulcer, as with almost all ulcers with a vasculitic component, is bluish-purple (b) due to haemorrhage within the skin. Associated diseases include inflammatory bowel disease, rheumatoid arthritis, paraproteinaemias and myeloproliferative disorders.

Fig. 12.3(a) shows multiple lesions of pyoderma gangrenosum in different stages of evolution, from the early red nodules and plaques to the purple-rimmed established ulcer. The characteristic histological features of pyoderma (i.e. heavy reutrophil infiltration of the dermis prior to ulceration) can only be seen in the red plaques and nodules. Once ulceration has occurred, it is difficult to distinguish histologically from other ulcers with a vasculitic pathogenesis (see (b)).

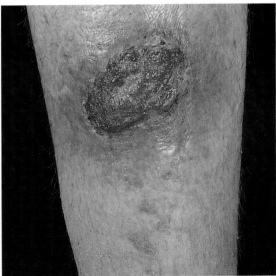

(b)

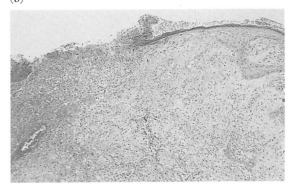

In the established ulcerated lesion of both pyoderma gangrenosum and other vasculitic ulcers there is a heavy, predominantly neutrophilic infiltrate in the dermis around the ulcer, which may be deep (c). Neutrophilic vasculitis is seen within the acute inflammatory zone around the ulcer crater, but the presence of vasculitis in the upper dermis at some distance from the active necrosis and inflammation suggests that the ulcerating lesion may have a vasculitic basis. This is supported by the observation of prominent neutrophilic vasculitis in the upper and mid-dermis in the early biopsy of non-ulcerated perilesional skin.

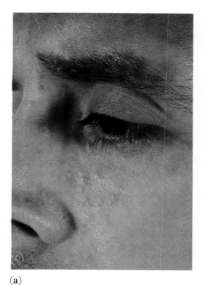

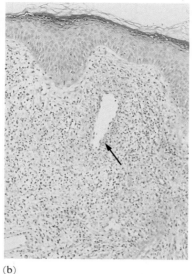

(a)

(b)

Fig. 12.4(a) & (b) Granuloma faciale

The usual history is of fleshy red or purple nodules on the face (a), or occasionally the trunk , which slowly but persistently enlarge. They are commonest in middle age. Although clinically they appear granulomatous, the histological appearances are more complex. There is a dense mixed inflammatory cell infiltrate of lymphocytes, histiocytes, plasma cells, eosinophils and some neutrophils in the upper and mid-dermis, but leaving a clear, uninvolved zone around skin appendages and beneath the epidermis. Within the inflammatory infiltrate may be found small vessels showing a neutrophilic vasculitis (arrow in (b)). This feature is more apparent in early lesions but becomes less obvious with the passage of time. A careful search should be made for vasculitis in any fixed facial eruption in which neutrophils and eosinophils are numerous.

LYMPHOCYTIC VASCULITIS

Lymphocytes appear in vessel walls at a late stage of what was originally a neutrophilic vasculitis, when they are usually part of a mixed inflammatory infiltrate of neutrophils, lymphocytes and histiocytes. True vasculitic lesions in which lymphocytes predominate throughout are rare, although perivascular lymphocytic infiltrates are extremely common in a wide range of inflammatory skin diseases. Careful histological examination is necessary when the inital impression is of a lymphocytic vasculitis to confirm that the lymphocytes are within the structures of the vessel wall. Accurate location of the lymphocytes is facilitated by the use of thin paraffin sections (2–3 µm), or acrylic resin sections (1–2 µm) if available. Rarely, leukaemic infiltrates (particularly in acute monocytic leukaemia) may mimic a lymphocytic vasculitis. A true lymphocytic infiltrate of vessel walls may occur in lymphomatoid papulosis and in the rare entity called lymphomatoid granulomatosis; the relationship between these two conditions and malignant lymphoma is discussed in Chapter 22. Lymphocytic infiltration of vessel walls should always raise suspicions of a lymphoma when the infiltrating lymphocytes will often be cytologically atypical, a feature best detected in acrylic resin sections. An extremely important (but often neglected) cause of lymphocytic vasculitis in the skin is in association with some of the connective tissue disorders. In this case the lymphocytes are not cytologically atypical, and there may be a small number of viable neutrophils or the pyknotic nuclear debris of dead neutrophils in the area, suggesting that there has been an earlier, transient phase of neutrophilic vasculitis. This is usually a cutaneous manifestation of a more generalized lymphocytic vasculitis, and there may be clinical and radiological evidence of lung involvement, and clinical and biochemical indications of skeletal muscle disease. Biopsies of muscle and lung may show similar lymphocytic vasculitis in these tissues.

As a general rule, a genuine lymphocytic vasculitis in the skin is an indication of a severe systemic disease, either immunological or lymphomatous, and merits detailed immunological and haematological investigation, although some drug reactions can show a mixture of lymphocytic vasculitis and 'toxic erythema' (see Fig. 14.1).

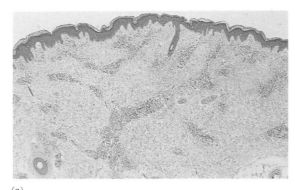

(a)

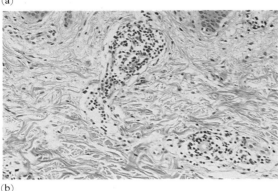

(b)

Fig. 12.5(a) & (b) Lymphocytic vasculitis
The clinical manifestations of mild lymphocytic vasculitis are often variable but in severe cases raised, reddish-purple plaques may be present resembling persistent chronic urticaria. The low power photomicrograph (a) shows such a severe case. Note that almost all the vessels in the mid- and upper dermis are apparently surrounded by a lymphocytic infiltrate. Closer histological examination, as in (b), shows that the infiltrate is not perivascular but is in fact invading the vessel wall and lymphocytes can be seen lining the lumen of the small vessel. Lymphocytic vasculitis of the degree demonstrated in micrograph (b) is often misdiagnosed as a perivascular lymphocytic infiltrate and its true significance is not appreciated.

Lymphocytic capillaritis

There are two conditions in which a *lymphocytic capillaritis* occurs in the upper dermis, but whether it is a primary or secondary phenomenon is not clear; these are pityriasis lichenoides et varioliformis acuta and the group of related disorders grouped under the name pigmented purpuric eruptions.

(a)

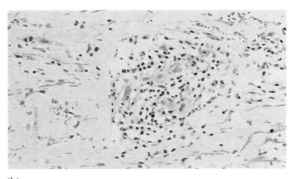

(b)

Fig. 12.6(a) & (b) Pigmented purpuric eruptions
This group of disorders appears to be due to an inflammatory capillaritis in the upper dermis. Capillaries are prominent and dilated, there is a lymphocytic infiltrate around the capillaries in the papillary dermis and some vessels show thickening and disruption of their walls with lymphocytes identifiable within the wall; endothelial cells are usually swollen and prominent. Associated with this histological evidence of capillaritis, there is visible extravasation of red blood cells into the loose papillary dermis; this is responsible for the clinically apparent purpura. Thus, the early lesions appear as patches of petechiae, usually on the lower trunk and lower limbs; however, with the passage of time the lesions change colour from red to brown, due to the formation of haemosiderin pigment in the upper dermis. This can be easily demonstrated by Perls stain. This combination of purpura and pigmentation is the basis for the name, pigmented purpuric eruption, but within this group are a number of eponymous disorders (e.g. Majocchi-Schamberg disease, Gougerot and Blum disease) all of which are best regarded as variants of a lymphocytic capillaritis, differing only in degree of telangiectasia and in secondary changes such as scaling, erythema, and lichenoid change.

HISTIOCYTIC VASCULITIS

The term granulomatous vasculitis is often inappropriately applied to this group because the histiocytic and giant cell aggregation, with the inflamed vessel at its centre, may produce a granuloma-like nodule. Furthermore, this pattern of vasculitis may occasionally be seen in association with a histiocytic granulomatous inflammation affecting the dermis and subcutis, e.g. in some cases of necrobiosis lipoidica. Many cases of histiocytic or granulomatous vasculitis begin as a neutrophilic vasculitis, but histiocytes and giant cells often dominate the picture at the time of biopsy, which is usually some time after the onset of the vasculitic process in the vessel wall. Histiocytic and giant cell infiltration is particularly likely to supervene when medium-sized or large arteries are involved, particularly those with a substantial elastin content. In vessels with a distinct elastic lamina, giant cells are particularly prominent in association with degenerate fragments of the elastic lamina. It can therefore be seen as a feature of polyarteritis nodosa and is particularly marked in some of its clinical variants such as Wegener's granulomatosis and Churg-Strauss allergic granulomatosis, as their names imply. Even the classical histiocytic and giant cell vasculitis, cranial or temporal arteritis, has an early neutrophilic vasculitic phase. Although not primarily a skin lesion, the commonly involved scalp vessels are subcutaneous and their occlusion can produce skin necrosis. An illustration is included here for completeness.

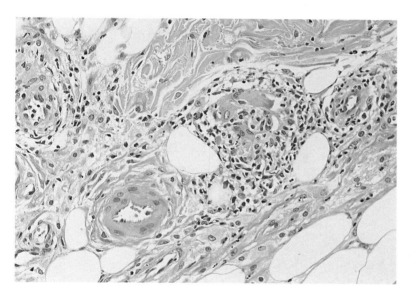

Fig. 12.7 Histiocytic (granulomatous) vasculitis
This skin vessel is from a patient with a systemic illness with some of the features of Churg-Strauss allergic granulomatosis and shows destruction of a vessel wall by lymphocytes, histiocytes and the formation of multinucleate giant cells. A few eosinophils are also present.

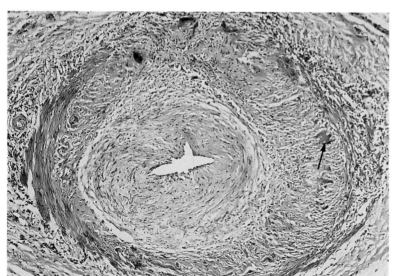

Fig. 12.8 Temporal arteritis at histiocytic/giant cell stage
This photomicrograph shows the typical features of temporal arteritis. The vessel wall is disrupted and shows a heavy infiltrate of lymphocytes and histiocytes and occasional multinucleate histiocytes (giant cells) are seen in association with the degenerated internal elastic lamina (arrow). Some neutrophils and eosinophils are also present. Note the great reduction in the size of the vessel lumen.

Inflammation of medium and large veins

Most of the clinically significant vasculitic disorders of the skin affect arteries, arterioles and capillaries, with occasional small venule involvement. However, inflammation of the walls of medium and large veins may occur in thrombophlebitis migrans and in the subcutaneous fat in some erythema nodosum lesions (see Fig 11.7).

Thrombosis in skin vessels

Any destructive vasculitis may be complicated by the formation of thrombus within the vessel lumen; this is particularly a feature of giant cell (temporal) arteritis and the small vessel neutrophilic vasculitis associated with meningococcal and gonococcal septicaemia. In these cases of secondary thrombosis, the vessels almost always show evidence of an active vasculitis, with a heavy vessel wall infiltrate of inflammatory cells and often fibrinoid necrosis of the walls. However, occasionally the thrombosis is extensive and the changes of inflammatory vasculitis are minor; this is particularly seen in disseminated intravascular coagulation of non-vasculitic origin, in cryoglobulinaemia, and in association with livedo reticularis and lupus anticoagulant, and acute meningococcal septicaemia.

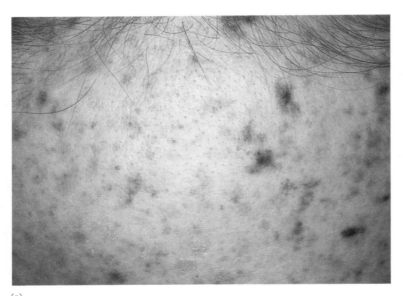

(a)

Fig. 12.9(a) & (b) Microvascular thrombosis in acute meningogoccal septicaemia
The extensive, rapidly spreading, purpuric and ecchymotic rash seen in fulminating meningococcal septicaemia is the result of widespread thrombosis in the small and medium vessels in the dermis and upper subcutis, with progressive extravasation of red blood cells. Histological evidence of vessel wall inflammation is usually minimal or absent. The clinical photograph (a) shows typical lesions on the forehead of a 17-year-old girl; elsewhere the lesions were ecchymotic and becoming confluent.

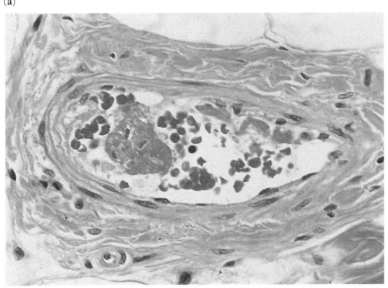

(b)

The photomicrograph(b) shows a small, thick-walled, upper dermal vessel which contains plugs of recently formed thrombus, composed of platelets and fibrin; around thinner-walled vessels there will be extravasation of red cells. Later lesions show larger masses of thrombus occluding the vessels and much more extensive extravasation of blood.

13. Mast cell disorders: urticaria and mastocytoses

Introduction

Mast cells are found in the connective tissue of most organs and are numerous in skin; they are frequently seen as a minority cell in many of the perivascular inflammatory cell infiltrates. Even in uninflamed skin, mast cells are mainly seen close to dermal blood vessels. Normally, they are round or oval cells with rather homogenous, purplish cytoplasm (on H & E staining) and a central or slightly eccentric, round, dark-staining nucleus; high resolution light microscopy of thin sections, particularly resin embedded, reveals fine cytoplasmic granules which are much easier to see in sections of all types when metachromatic staining methods, such as Toluidine Blue, are used. The granules have a characteristic electron-dense, lamellated appearance on electron microscopy. They contain heparin and histamine, as well as a number of other chemical mediators; release occurs following interaction of antigen with IgE bound to the mast cell membrane, but can also occur non-immunologically. This release is usually associated with degranulation of the mast cells, and the various released substances cause increased vascular permeability, fluid transudation, and activation of platelets and eosinophils. Clinically this all results in urticaria, i.e. localized dermal oedema with severe itch. In the mastocytoses, mast cells are present in greatly increased numbers; in the commonest, proliferation is confined to skin. Lesions may be single (mastocytoma) or multiple (urticaria pigmentosa). Systemic involvement can occur rarely, with lesions in many organs, particularly the bone marrow and spleen.

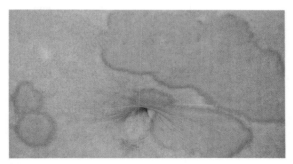

(a)

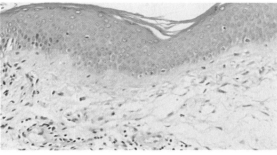

(b)

Fig. 13.1(a) & (b). Acute urticaria

Urticaria is extremely common, and is usually easily diagnosed clinically. Lesions begin as red papules which often within 10–30 minutes develop into 0.5–3 cm pale wheals with a surrounding red flare, which usually disappears within 1–12 hours (a). Involvement of subcutaneous tissue (angioedema), especially around the mouth and eyes, also occurs. Usually the cause is unclear but less commonly, urticaria can be provoked by sweating (cholinergic urticaria), heat, sunlight, cold, pressure (physical urticaria). Papular urticaria is due to insect bites and usually occurs seasonally in children. H1 blockade sufficient to inhibit histamine whealing is usually effective treatment but often fails to completely suppress chronic idiopathic urticaria, suggesting that other mediators are involved. More persistent urticarial lesions lasting several days may be due to skin vasculitis, especially if resulting in bruising.

Histologically, the changes are not dramatic, the most obvious feature being oedema in all layers of the dermis, separating the individual bundles of collagen fibres; the papillary dermis is usually less affected than the reticular dermis. Despite the fact that mast cells are responsible for the reaction, they are extremely sparse, just a few being found mixed with eosinophils and scanty lymphocytes around some dermal vessels, which usually show dilatation and associated endothelial cell swelling. Although most acute urticarial lesions are usually transient, more persistent lesions (b) show a more abundant perivascular inflammatory cell infiltrate and involvement of the papillary dermis.

In papular urticaria the papules show a localized area of perivascular infiltrate with lymphocytes, histiocytes, eosinophils and mast cells in the upper dermis, with variable oedema between collagen fibres, and a light scattering of eosinophils and mast cells away from vessels in the upper and mid-dermis. In the epidermis overlying the most marked and superficial perivascular infiltrate, the epidermis shows spongiosis with exocytosis and vesicle formation. In older excoriated lesions, the histological changes are usually modified by the effects of scratching, with the development of epidermal necrosis, crusting and dermal infiltrate with neutrophils and more abundant lymphocytes, making histological diagnosis difficult. Excoriated or scratched lesions should not be biopsied.

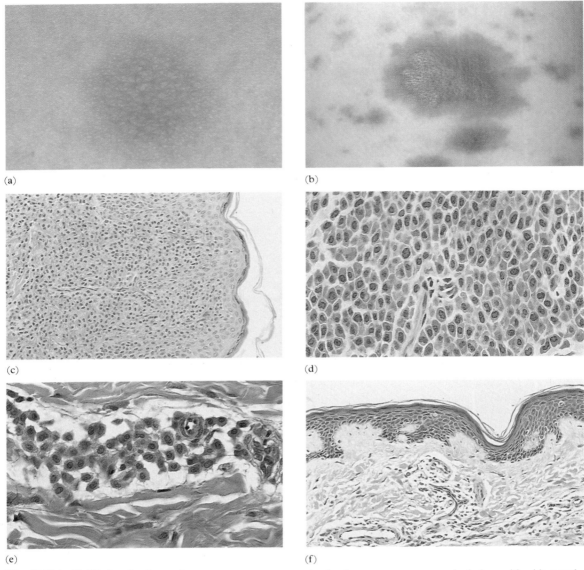

(a)

(b)

(c)

(d)

(e)

(f)

Fig. 13.2(a)–(f). Urticaria pigmentosa

This is a spectrum of disorders in which persistent mast cell accumulation in the skin is a common feature. Characteristically, lesions will urticate after rubbing, becoming itchy, and surrounded by a red flare. They are variably pigmented with melanin. Stroking non-lesional skin produces a wheal with an irregular edge (beaded dermographism) due to focal populations of mast cells.

The following patterns are recognized:

1. **Solitary mastocytoma** (a): largely confined to infants, this presents as a 1–3 cm red or brown oval lesion usually appearing in the first few months of life on the trunk or limbs. They are nearly always self-limiting, and blistering due to dermo-epidermal separation is common.

2. **Multiple lesions** (b): these lesions are smaller, usually macules, papules and nodules, but are similarly red or brown in colour. They are often very widespread, especially on the trunk, and are commonest in children when they are usually self-limiting. Adult disease may

develop into, or appear as, macular lesions with widespread persistent telangiectasia (telangiectasia macularis eruptiva perstans). Rarely, a diffuse mast cell infiltration of the skin is accompanied by the developement of systemic lesions, and systemic histamine release can occur, with flushing, bronchospasm and hypotension.

Figures 13.2(c) and (d) show the histological appearances of a solitary mastocytoma in which mast cells form a tumour-like mass in the upper dermis; see also Figure 2.5(a). Photomicrograph (e) shows the maculopapular type in which the mast cells are scattered more diffusely through the upper dermis to form a macule with occasional packed aggregates producing small papules; (f) shows the macular telangiectatic variant in which the major histological feature is prominent thick-walled and dilated dermal blood vessels, and mast cells are usually scanty and mainly concentrated around the abnormal blood vessels.

14. Skin eruptions due to ingested drugs

Introduction

Drug-induced skin lesions are becoming more frequent and diverse in pattern as the repertoire of pharmacological agents increases and drugs are more widely prescribed. Clinical diagnosis is always easier than histological diagnosis, for there are no histological features pathognomonic of drug-induced change and the history is paramount.

The following clinical features may help in diagnosis:

1. Some drugs are unlikely to cause rashes, e.g. digoxin, anticoagulants, benzodiazepines.

2. Drug rashes usually develop at least 7 days after first exposure, recur within 20 days of re-exposure, and improve within 3–4 days of stopping the drug. There are a number of important exceptions, for example, the rapid onset of erythema nodosum and/or multiforme with cotrimoxazole, and the very slow resolution of erythroderma after captopril.

3. Skin rashes rarely occur as a result of intravenous drug therapy; an important exception is the widespread allergic dermatitis which may follow intravenous aminophylline in patients with prior cutaneous sensitization to ethylenediamine which is present in some topical applications.

4. In rashes due to allergic mechanisms (the majority), there is probably an inverse relationship between duration of drug exposure and incidence of rashes, but increasing exposure or dose increases risk if the mechanism is pharmacological. Both allergic and pharmacological mechanisms can operate.

Classification of skin eruptions

Skin eruptions due to drugs can be considered under the following headings:

1. Toxic erythemas;
2. Erythema multiforme and toxic epidermal necrolysis;
3. Lichen planus and lichenoid eruptions;
4. Urticarial eruptions;
5. Purpuric reactions;
6. Photosensitivity dermatitis;
7. Fixed drug eruption;
8. Miscellaneous reactions.

Toxic erythemas

Toxic erythemas are the most common pattern of drug reaction, but are not specific and can also occur for other reasons, e.g. associated with viraemia (such as the 'slapped cheek syndrome' associated with parvovirus infection) or bacterial toxins. Erythema is the term used to describe varying degrees of reddening of the skin. In simple erythema the skin is diffusely red, partly due to vasodilatation, and hence blanches on pressure. Occasionally, severe toxic erythema becomes an *erythroderma*, and becomes indistinguishable in appearance from other causes of erythroderma such as psoriasis. Erythroderma is the term used to describe widespread erythema affecting virtually the entire skin surface; it may be followed by extensive scaling (exfoliative

Table 14.1 Common causes of erythroderma

Cause	Clinical	Pathological features
Drug reaction e.g. gold, carbamezepine sulphonamides' captopril	History	Toxic erythema, exocytosis
Psoriasis	Previous psoriasis	Psoriatic features histologically
Atopic and seborrhoeic dermatitis	Particularly infants and elderly	Non-specific dermatitis
Pityriasis rubra pilaris	Small patches of normal pale skin	Follicular plugging and parakeratosis
Cutaneous T cell lymphoma	Sézary syndrome lymphadenopathy	Malignant T cell infiltrate
Leukaemia (chronic lymphocytic)	Blood film and bone marrow	Leukaemic infiltrate in dermis

dermatitis). Histological features vary according to the cause, but upper dermal vascular dilatation and lymphocyte infiltration is a constant finding. Important causes of erythroderma are summarized in Table 14.1.

Drugs which produce toxic erythemas include antibiotics (especially ampicillin and sulphonamides), barbiturates and chlorpropamide.

Erythema multiforme and toxic epidermal necrolysis

Erythema multiforme may be precipitated by a number of factors, including drugs. It has a number of clinical patterns, ranging from irregular patches of erythema of many shapes and sizes (multiforme), to discrete annular target lesions with or without central blisters, to extensive blistering and ulcerating lesions affecting skin and mucous membranes (blistering erythema multiforme or Stevens-Johnson syndrome; see Fig. 14.3). The most severe form is an extensive blistering lesion, often originating in the mucosa but shortly manifesting in the skin flexures such as the axillae and groin but ultimately involving much of the body surface; this is called *toxic epidermal necrolysis* and, like the Stevens-Johnson syndrome, is much more likely to have a drug aetiology than other, milder, forms of erythema multiforme.

The clinical and histological features of the various patterns of erythema multiforme are illustrated in Figures 14.2, 14.3 and 14.4 in this chapter, and in Figure 8.7 in the chapter on blistering disorders.

Lichen planus and lichenoid eruptions

The clinical and pathological features of lichen planus are discussed and illustrated in Chapter 7. Although most cases are of unknown aetiology, a proportion follow ingestion of certain drugs such as methyldopa, gold and penicillamine. Such cases are clinically and histologically identical to spontaneous lichen planus, but tend to resolve more quickly once the drug has been stopped.

Urticarial eruptions

Urticaria is discussed and illustrated in Chapter 13. Drug-induced urticaria differs little from spontaneous urticaria (see Fig. 13.1) in its clinical appearance, but the presence of occasional neutrophils and eosinophils around upper and mid-dermal vessels should raise the possibility of a drug aetiology. This type of histological appearance is sometimes called an urticarial allergic eruption to distinguish it from the more common type of urticaria which is comparatively devoid of cellular infiltrate. A history of drug ingestion, e.g. penicillin, may precede an attack, but often the patient does not admit a drug history. Since aspirin may precipitate urticaria it is worth enquiring about the taking of proprietary analgesics and 'cold-cures'.

Purpuric reactions

Although clinically there is sometimes a purpuric element to the drug-induced erythemas, some drugs, e.g. certain sulphonamides, can produce a pure purpuric rash which is histologically based on an acute neutrophilic vasculitis affecting small upper dermal vessels; see Figure 12.1(b) and (c). It is not possible to distinguish this from other causes of acute neutrophilic vasculitis (see Ch. 12) on histological grounds, but a disproportionate number of eosinophils, and specific involvement of very small upper dermal vessels, are pointers to a drug aetiology.

Photosensitivity dermatitis

Some drugs, such as frusemide, sulphonamides, phenothiazines, tetracyclines, act as photosensitizers in that they can produce skin rashes in susceptible people by interaction with ultraviolet light. An erythematous rash or an acute dermatitis occurs in skin exposed to quite moderate amounts of sunlight, the impression being of inappropriately severe sunburn.

Histologically, there is capillary dilatation in the upper dermis, with a scanty perivascular lymphocytic infiltrate. The epidermis contains scattered necrotic keratinocytes, mainly near the surface, but there may also be necrosis of some basal cells with hydropic degeneration in others; in severe lesions there may be basal blistering. The changes somewhat resemble those of mild erythema multiforme (see Fig. 14.2).

Fixed drug eruption

This term is used to describe a clinically distinct reaction to drug ingestion in which the lesion occurs at the same site with subsequent exposures to the drug. The clinical and histological features are illustrated in Figure 14.5.

Miscellaneous drug-related eruptions

In addition to the conditions described above, there are a number of skin disorders which can occasionally be initiated by drugs. Erythema nodosum (see Fig. 11.7) may be induced by sulphonamide or antibiotic therapy, discoid dermatitis (see Fig. 5.7) by gold and methyldopa, and acneiform folliculitis (see Fig. 10.12) by corticosteroids and progestogens. Eruptions which closely resemble spontaneously occurring skin disease can also be associated with drugs, although they have a different natural history, usually responding quickly or slowly to removal of the drug. Examples include the pemphigus vulgaris-like lesion or the CTCL-like lesions associated with captopril, and pemphigus vulgaris or vegetans with penicillamine.

EXAMPLES OF SPECIFIC DRUG REACTIONS

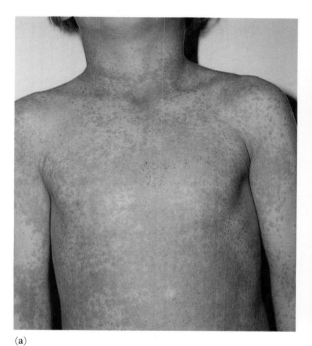

(a)

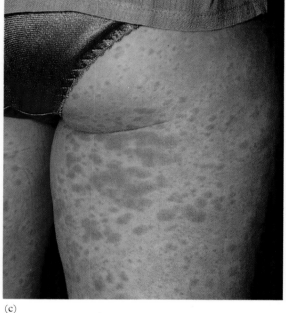

(c)

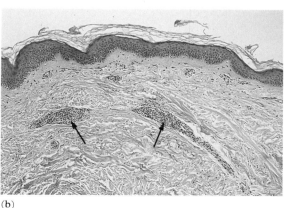

(b)

Fig. 14.1(a), (b) & (c) Toxic erythema
The most frequent clinical appearance is of a red macular rash which becomes papular (a), the individual lesions becoming confluent to form a widespread blotchiness with surface desquamation.

Histologically, the characteristic feature is a compact lymphocytic infiltrate around upper dermal vessels (arrows). The infiltrate is particularly widespread but very closely confined to the region immediately around the vessels (b) and there is little or no extension of the infiltrate into dermal connective tissue. The affected vessels may be dilated and have prominent swollen endothelial cells. In papular or urticarial erythematous lesions, the changes are accompanied by some dermal oedema; the example illustrated in (c) is a drug reaction to a non-steroidal anti-inflammatory drug. In such raised lesions with urticarial features, there may be a lymphocytic vasculitis (see p. 105 and Fig. 12.5); it is important to examine such lesions at high magnification to differentiate it from a perivascular lymphocytic infiltrate.

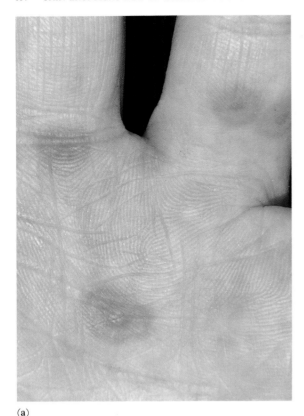

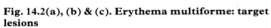

(a)

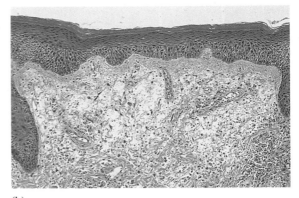

(b)

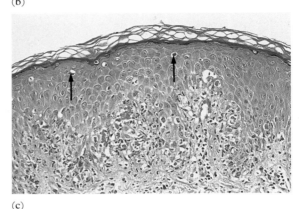

(c)

Fig. 14.2(a), (b) & (c). Erythema multiforme: target lesions

The clinical photograph shows a typical target lesion of erythema multiforme situated on the hands which is a common site. This pattern of lesion is also commonly seen on the forearms, feet and lower legs, and occasionally on the external genitalia. Note the well-circumscribed red lesions with central vesicle formation.

Histologically, the raised red peripheral area shows oedema and lymphocytic infiltrate in the upper dermis, the infiltrate being particularly concentrated around the vessels, and the oedema most marked in the papillae(b). Micrograph (c) shows vacuolar hydropic degeneration of basal cells, associated with exocytosis of inflammatory cells; this change is most marked in the centre of the lesion where there is

early separation of epidermis from dermis to form a small sub-epidermal vesicle which may enlarge to form a clinically obvious blister. A characteristic feature of erythema multiforme of any pattern is the presence of necrotic eosinophilic keratinocytes both in the basal and spinous layers, as indicated by the arrows in micrograph (c). In lesions such as this, they may be few and scattered, being most obvious in the basal layers at the periphery of the blister and in the prickle cell layer forming the roof of the blister. Epidermal cell necrosis is extensive in the more severe widespread blistering lesions, where the change is responsible for enlargement of the blister by adding an intra-epidermal blister component to the already established sub-epidermal blister. An example of blistering erythema multiforme is illustrated in Figure 14.3.

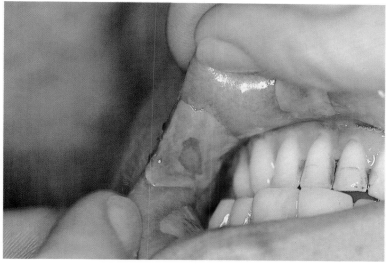

(a)

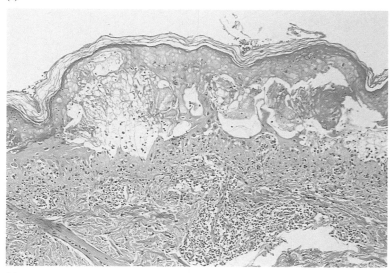

(b)

Fig. 14.3(a) & (b). Blistering erythema multiforme

Clinically, the most severe lesions in erythema multiforme present as large blisters, followed by painful erosions on mucosal surfaces, as in the buccal lesions shown here (a). Note the pale membrane of necrotic mucosal epithelium still adherent, with central erosion. It is sometimes called the Stevens-Johnson syndrome. Usual causes are infections (especially herpes simplex) and drugs (especially penicillin).

Histologically, there is characteristic necrosis of epidermal cells, usually scattered in the basal and prickle cell layers, associated with varying degrees of blister formation. Most blisters arise at the basal region to form a subepidermal bulla which is roofed by epidermis in which there is focal necrosis of epidermal cells. Basal cell necrosis is extensive, leading to large subepidermal bullae, and the roof of epidermis shows widespread necrosis affecting almost all cells (b); dissolution of the necrotic roof produces extensive areas of raw superficial oozing. When the blister is intact, its fluid contains lymphocytes and necrotic epidermal cells, and the base is dermis containing a lymphocytic inflammatory cell infiltrate. Another pattern of blister formation is often seen in association with the basal blistering described above: in addition to the pattern of basal cell necrosis, there are often areas of ballooning degeneration of epidermal cells, continued breakdown of which leads to reticular degeneration of the epidermis with the formation of intra-epidermal blisters as here. Again the roof of the blister is often composed of necrotic upper epidermis.

Fig. 14.4(a), (b) & (c). Toxic epidermal necrolysis (TEN)

This is best regarded as a severe variant of blistering erythema multiforme in which the major lesion is in the epidermis; drugs are the usual cause. Clinically, spreading erythema is rapidly followed by flaccid blistering and shedding of large sheets of necrotic epidermis, leaving a red, oozing, denuded surface which is naked dermis (a). There is loss of appendages and severe involvement of mucosal surfaces. Separation of apparently uninvolved epidermis by shearing is also seen (Nikolsky's sign). Even before any secondary infection of exposed dermis by bacteria, or electrolyte imbalance due to fluid and salt loss from the surface, the patient shows evidence of severe systemic illness with fever and shock. Clinically, it is usually distinguishable from staphylococcal scalded skin syndrome in children: in toxic epidermal necrolysis freshly separated skin is composed of the full thickness epidermis, and so frozen sections can sometimes provide a rapid answer.

In the established lesion there is extensive epidermal cell necrosis and complete separation of epidermis from dermis. The floor of the blister is formed by naked dermis in which there is usually a very scanty lymphocytic infiltrate (b). In some cases of drug-induced disease there may be a few eosinophils. The blister is usually flaccid, containing little fluid and virtually no cells, the necrotic epidermal roof being shed before any pressure builds up, leaving denuded oozing dermis. Dermal inflammation is therefore usually less marked in TEN than it is in other blistering forms of erythema multiforme but is more prominent at the margins of the blistering area and in erythematous patches where separation has not occurred. In these areas, ballooning degeneration and individual cell necrosis are frequent in basal cells and in scattered prickle cells (c), but once separation occurs the entire sheet of epidermis roofing the blister is usually necrotic. At an early stage, when the lesion is clinically in the form of a spreading erythema, the histological changes are similar to those seen at the edge of the blistering area, i.e. individual foci of epidermal necrosis associated with oedema of the upper dermis with inflammatory cell infiltrate and mild exocytosis.

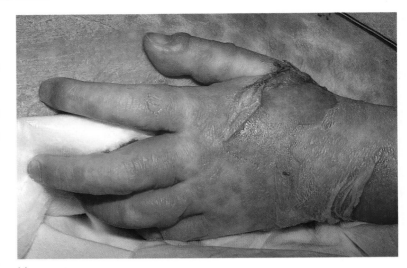

(a)

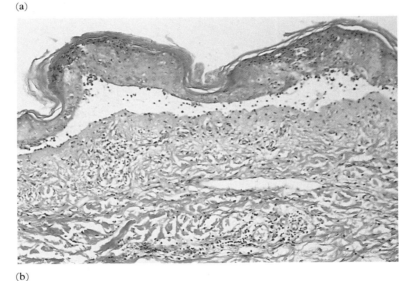

(b)

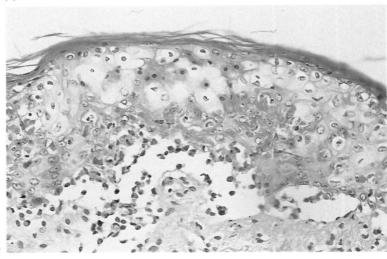

(c)

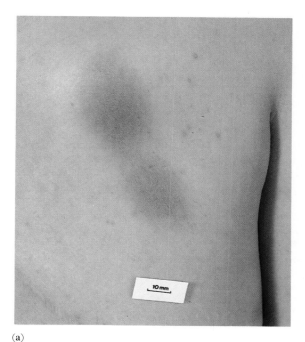

(a)

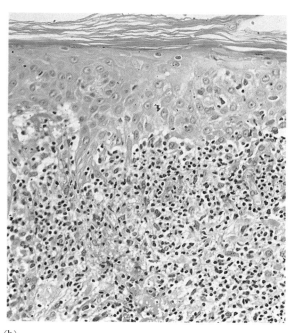

(b)

Fig. 14.5(a) & (b). Fixed drug eruption

This presents as one or several raised oedematous or indurated reddish-brown plaques, usually roughly rounded, often on the face, upper trunk or limbs (a); it arises shortly after ingestion of the causative drug and recurs at the same site if the drug is given again. Occasionally, the centre of the raised plaque shows bulla formation. With cessation of the drug, the lesion subsides quickly, leaving a circumscribed patch of increased melanin pigmentation. Histologically, the lesion shows features resembling erythema multiforme. There is variable dermal oedema (responsible for the elevation of the lesion) and dilatation of upper dermal vessels, many of which have a lymphocytic infiltrate around them, the dilatation and infiltrate together producing the red coloration of the plaque. In early lesions there may be a few neutrophils and eosinophils in the perivascular infiltrate. In the upper dermis the inflammatory cells spread into the connective tissues of the papillae and begin to encroach into lower layers of the epidermis (exocytosis) which shows hydropic degeneration and focal epidermal cell necrosis (b). When basal cell damage and epidermal cell necrosis are severe, a bulla forms, the roof of which is often greyish in colour, the result of necrosis of the superficial epidermal cells.

As the lesion resolves, the inflammatory cell infiltrate becomes less and the epidermal damage dies down. As the inflammatory infiltrate diminishes, the plaque becomes flatter until it reaches the level of surrounding skin. If there has been significant basal cell damage, the resolved lesion will appear hyperpigmented as a result of residual melanin-laden macrophages (melanophages) remaining in the upper dermis long after the other components of the upper dermal inflammatory cell infiltrate have largely disappeared; the melanin is derived from the damaged basal cells and melanocytes. Even in a plaque which is still active, dermal melanin gives a reddish-brown color to the lesion, the degree of brownness giving some indication of the severity of the basal layer damage. With continuing resolution the redness fades and the lesion becomes brown. At this late stage, the lesion is histologically indistinguishable from many other resolving skin conditions which, in their active phase, are characterized by extensive basal cell damage. Obviously, the greater the original degree of skin pigmentation, the greater the degree of postinflammatory hyperpigmentation.

Histological diagnosis of drug reactions

Although drugs can produce almost any pattern of skin lesion, it is of little value to clinicians for the pathologist to suggest a diagnosis of drug reaction for every biopsy which does not fit into a well-recognized diagnostic group. In any case, the dermatologist is usually in a better position than the pathologist to assess whether a skin eruption is likely to be drug-related. Listed below are a few useful pointers which should alert the pathologist to a drug aetiology:

1. A histologically distinct pattern occurring in an inappropriate site, age group or circumstance; for example, a lesion with the features of herpes gestationis occurring in an elderly man.

2. Very sharply defined perivascular cuffing with lymphocytes in all layers of the dermis, in lesions described as being erythematous clinically.

3. An unusual predominance of eosinophils in perivascular inflammatory infiltrates.

4. Confinement of acute neutrophilic vasculitis to very small vessels in the upper dermis.

15. Disorders of dermal fibres and ground substance

Introduction

The normal dermis is described and illustrated in Chapter 3 (Fig. 3.15); its structural integrity and resistance to injury result from its collagen and elastic fibres, and the mucopolysaccharide ground substance in which they are embedded. Abnormalities in these three components alter the appearance and texture of the skin. The thinning and fragility of the skin seen in elderly people is largely due to collagen loss and alterations in the nature of the elastic fibres.

There are many skin conditions in which the major abnormality is in the quality or quantity of dermal fibres (collagen and elastin) or ground substance (acid mucopolysaccharides syn glycosaminoglycans), and a small group in which various substances are deposited in the dermis to produce clinically visible abnormalities. A simple classification of disorders of dermal fibres and ground substance is given below:

Changes in quantity or quality of dermal fibres

Scar
Keloid
Solar elastosis   See this chapter
Lichen sclerosus et atrophicus
Pseudoxanthoma elasticum
Ehlers Danlos syndrome

Granuloma annulare   These disorders are associated with the development of a
Necrobiosis lipoidica   granulomatous tissue reaction to collagen degeneration and
Rheumatoid nodule   are dealt with in Chapter 11.

Scleroderma/morphoea   These are illustrated and discussed in Chapter 9.

Changes in ground substance
Pretibial myxoedema
Lichen myxoedematosus/scleromyxoedema   See this chapter
Scleroedema

Depositions in dermis
Amyloid   See this chapter
Calcinosis cutis

Gout   Urate crystals excite a florid granulomatous reaction and
                                   gout is illustrated in Chapter 11

CHANGES IN DERMAL FIBRES

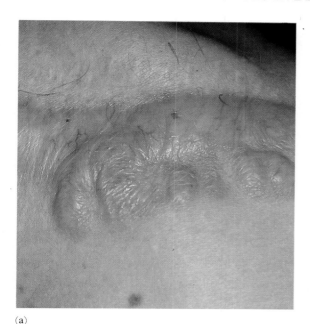

(a)

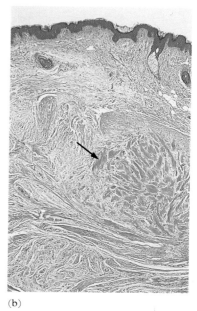

(b)

Fig. 15.1(a) & (b). Hypertrophic scar and keloid
Fibroblastic proliferation and collagen formation in the
dermis are vital components of the repair process following
damage to the skin. Under normal circumstances, the slow
growth of such fibrocollagenous tissue leads to a scar.
Occasionally, there is increased proliferation of fibroblasts
and collagen deposition, leading to the fomation of either a
hypertrophic scar which involutes, or a *keloid* which doesn't.

Keloids have a characteristic appearance. They can
develop within 2–3 weeks of injury, usually in adolescents,
particularly negroes, and at sites such as ears, shoulders and
central chest and back; the scar evolves into a red,
smooth-surfaced, domed, telangiectatic plaque (a). In the

illustrated example the lesion on the shoulder shows the
characteristic features of a surgical scar with keloid
formation at the site of the scar. They initially have a
regular outline but continued growth may produce a ragged
edge and persistence characteristic of keloid; scars which are
merely hypertrophic involute within several months. Both
show similar histological appearances, in that the dermis
contains large nodules of dense eosinophilic collagen made
up of whorls in which the collagen is densely compacted and
appears hyalinized (arrow in (b)). In keloids, these masses
persist and even enlarge, whereas in hypertrophic scars they
gradually involute, leaving collagen fibres orientated in the
way in which they normally lie in a reparative scar in the skin.

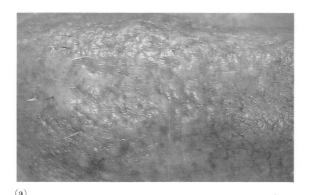

(a)

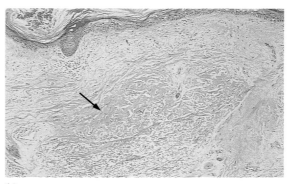

(b)

Fig. 15.2(a) & (b). Solar elastosis
This is due to disintegration of dermal collagen and elastin
after prolonged exposure to sunlight, mainly in fair-skinned
elderly people. The physical signs are ill-defined yellowish
cobble-stone plaques, often over the forehead and temples,
with telangiectasia (a). The histological characteristics are a
peculiar basophilic degeneration of upper dermis (arrow),

separated from the thinned epidermis by a narrow zone of
normal collagen (b). The amorphous purplish-staining
material shows some of the staining characteristics of
elastin, and appears to replace normal dermal collagen.
Occasionally, large nodules of this elastotic material occur
and this may be associated with cystically dilated hair
follicles and comedones.

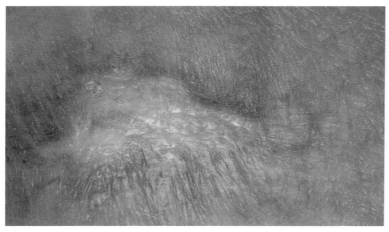

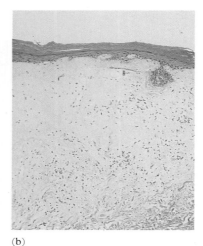

(a)

(b)

Fig. 15.3(a) & (b). Lichen sclerosus et atrophicus

This occurs most commonly in middle-aged and elderly women, mainly around the vulva and anus, but is also found on the glans penis and foreskin in men (balanitis xerotica obliterans). Lesions may also occur extragenitally on neck, trunk and limbs, and particularly on the flexor aspects of the wrists. The lesions begin as white shiny angular papules which coalesce into plaques (a). Follicular keratotic plugs are common, giving the lesion a rough surface; in early lesions, hyperkeratosis of the entire surface is frequent. The white colour is due to this, as well as to loss of melanin and presence of dermal oedema, and the 'waxy' feel is the result of subsequent atrophy. Subsequently, the overlying epidermis thins and telangiectasia may be visible. Histologically, the main abnormality is dermal; there is oedema and homogenization of collagen in the upper dermis, beneath which is a lymphocytic infiltrate in all but the oldest lesions. The oedematous upper dermis contains

prominent dilated blood vessels, responsible for the telangiectasia easily visible through the thinned epidermis which often shows hyperkeratosis (b). Because the lesions are itchy, secondary traumatic changes are sometimes seen. The dermal swelling, combined with the epidermal atrophy, leads to reduction in size and number of rete ridges, rendering the area prone to subepidermal bulla formation and haemorrhage when subjected to shearing stress such as rubbing.

Early indication of incipient epidermal separation is the appearance of basal cell hydropic degeneration and focally severe subepidermal oedema. Occasionally, in long-standing, chronically irritated lesions around the vulva and anus, there may be some focal acanthosis. In some such lesions the epidermis may also show moderate or severe dysplasia, and the development of invasive squamous carcinoma can occur in long-neglected lesions. This is a less frequent complication of extragenital skin lesions.

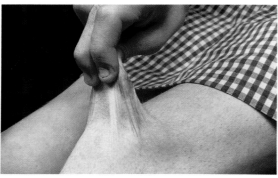

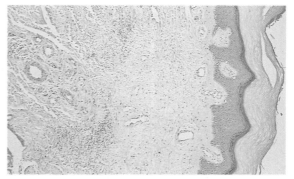

(a)

(b)

Fig. 15.4(a) & (b). Ehlers Danlos Syndrome

This is one of a group of inherited disorders of collagen synthesis in which collagen is abnormal in many of the areas of the body. Skin manifestations are a characteristic hyperelasticity (a) (in which the skin returns to normal when released), skin fragility with easy bruising, and impaired healing after injury, resulting in large, unsightly atrophic scars. Traumatic haematomas sometimes form in the dermis and subcutis, and resolve incompletely, leaving a raised fleshy lump, one of which is visible just below the patient's index finger in the clinical photograph. By light

microscopy, undamaged skin appears normal, although scanning electron microscopy has revealed abnormal organization of collagen fibrils in some cases.

The nodular masses which persist after haematoma formation are irregular masses of vascular fibrous tissue (b) containing some macrophages and giant cells in which haemosiderin has accumulated.

Systemic manifestations include hyperextensibility of joints, frequent dislocation, osteoarthritis and, in some variants, dissecting aneurysms.

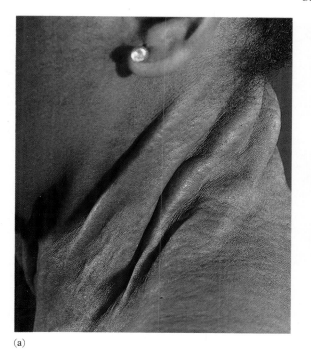

(a)

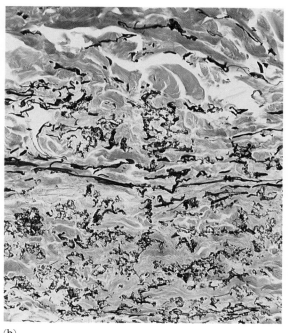

(b)

Fig. 15.5(a) & (b). Pseudoxanthoma elasticum
This is a rare group of inherited disorders of elastic fibre
formation. The skin manifestations are the development of
yellowish papules on the sides and back of the neck, usually
in early adult life. With the passage of time these enlarge
and become confluent and the affected skin becomes loose,
wrinkled and thickened. Changes may also be seen in the
axillae and groins, antecubital and popliteal fossae, and
around the umbilicus; retinal angioid streaks are also
characteristic. Elastic fibres in systemic blood vessels are
also affected, and there is an increased risk of coronary
artery disease, gastrointestinal tract and retinal

haemorrhage, and renovascular hypertension. *Perforating
elastoma* is also associated , in which yellowish plaques of
inelastic thickened skin are surrounded by papules with
central holes through which material is discharged.

The histological features are characteristic; the elastic
fibres in the mid- and lower dermis are increased in
number, but are short, thick, fragmented and wrinkled or
coiled. These abnormal fibres are easily seen in a routine
haematoxylin and eosin stain because they stain faintly blue
or purple, probably due to calcium deposition. They are
best demonstrated by an elastic tissue stain such as the
elastic-van Gieson stain shown here (b).

CHANGES IN GROUND SUBSTANCE

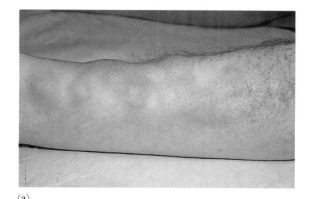

(a)

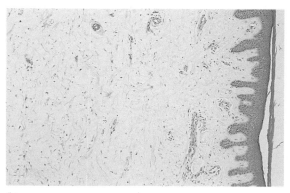

(b)

Fig. 15.6(a) & (b). Pretibial myxoedema
This lesion is associated with autoimmune thyrotoxicosis
and comprises pale flesh-coloured raised plaques on the
anterior shins, with a 'peau d'orange' surface, occasionally
extending onto the dorsa of the feet, and round the

calves (a).

The dermis is expanded by large quantities of
mucinous ground substance, mainly in mid-dermis (b),
separating the collagen bundles, often into separate fibres.
The ground substance is strongly Alcian blue positive.

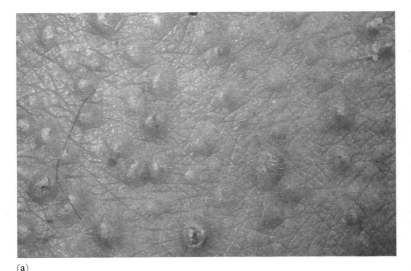

(a)

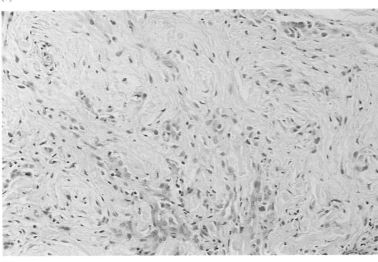

(b)

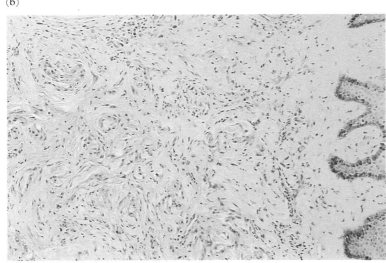

(c)

Fig. 15.7(a), (b) & (c). Lichen myxoedematosus and scleromyxoedema
These two conditions are histologically similar but have clinically distinct patterns. Both show excessive deposition of acid mucopolysaccharide ground substance between existing collagen fibres in the upper and mid-reticular dermis, but differ from pretibial myxoedema by the presence of proliferation of fibroblasts. Clinically, lichen myxoedematosus appears as numerous minute soft papules on the face, arms and sometimes upper trunk (a), whereas in scleromyxoedema the papular rash is accompanied by a diffuse thickening and induration of the skin, sometimes with erythema. Photomicrograph (b) stained by haematoxylin and eosin shows the material occupying the dermis to be lamellar mucinous material intermixed with some inflammatory cells and proliferating fibroblasts. Photomicrograph (c) stained by the Alcian blue method shows excessive amounts of Alcian blue positive mucinous ground substance interspersed with the nuclei of proliferating fibroblasts and some inflammatory cells, largely confined to reticular dermis.

Both disorders are associated in most cases with a monoclonal gammopathy, and in some patients a co-existent myeloma is discovered.

Scleroedema is a condition in which there is diffuse swelling and hardening of the skin, usually commencing on the face and spreading to the neck and upper trunk. Lesions associated with diabetes mellitus are persistent and unresponsive to treatment. The skin changes are due to a combination of collagenous replacement of adipose tissue in subcutaneous fat, and increased acid mucopolysaccharide ground substance between dermal collagen bundles. *Reticular erythematous mucinosis* is a rare condition in which there is increase in dermal acid mucopolysaccharides associated with a chronic inflammatory cell infiltrate around dermal blood vessels and hair follicles. It presents as clearly defined irregular erythematous plaques, usually on the chest or back, often appearing to form by confluence of multiple papules. The excessive acid mucopolysaccharide ground substance is particularly prominent in early papules.

In *follicular mucinosis*, the increase in acid mucopolysaccharides is most obvious in degenerate hair follicles, but there is also an increase in the dermis, in association with the invariable mixed inflammatory infiltrate. As a possible precursor of CTCL, this disorder is discussed and illustrated in Chapter 24.

Localized dermal mucinous accumulations are seen in *focal mucinosis* and *digital mucous cyst*.

DEPOSITIONS IN DERMIS

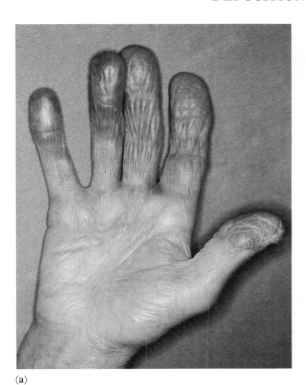

(a)

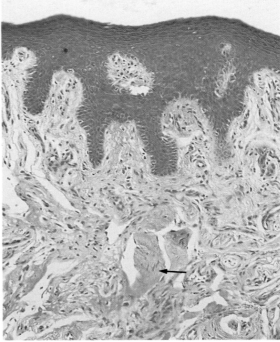

(b)

Fig. 15.8(a) & (b) Amyloid in skin

Significant amyloid deposition in the skin occurs most frequently in so-called 'primary' amyloidosis, although electron microscopy may reveal amyloid fibrils within the walls of dermal blood vessels and in the interstitium of subcutaneous fat in many cases of systemic amyloidosis, irrespective of type. Common clinical manifestations are petechiae and ecchymoses, particularly on the face, sometimes following minimal trauma. These result from the increased fragility of dermal blood vessels infiltrated by amyloid. There may also be rather waxy papules or plaques (a), the result of deposition of amyloid masses in the upper dermis.

In addition to cutaneous involvement in systemic amyloidosis, there are forms in which the amyloid deposition is confined to skin and there is no evidence of systemic involvement. They present either as groups of itchy/red-brown papules with surface scale, often on the legs (lichenoid amyloidosis) or as itchy macules showing reticulate brown pigmentation, often on the back (macular amyloidosis). The two patterns may co-exist, or there may be transition from one to the other, particularly from macular to lichenoid forms. The lesions are the result of deposition of amyloid in the papillary dermis, immediately beneath the epidermis. In the macular pattern the deposits may be small, and special staining methods (e.g. Congo Red) or even electron microscopy may be required to demonstrate them; in the lichenoid pattern the masses are more substantial and are usually easily seen in routine H & E sections (arrow in (b)). Acanthosis and hyperkeratosis are usual in lichenoid amyloidosis.

Fig. 15.9(a) & (b). Calcinosis cutis
Some cases of calcium deposition in
the skin are secondary to disordered
calcium or phosphate matabolism
(e.g. hyperparathyroidism or renal
osteodystrophy), whereas in others, the
calcium deposition occurs as a
secondary change in tissues previously
damaged (e.g. in progressive systemic
sclerosis). In the remainder, no
obvious predisposing factor is
identified (idiopathic calcinosis cutis).
The most common site is the scrotum,
where the lesions present as variably
sized, hard, yellowish-white nodules
which slowly enlarge over the years;
they may be present in childhood but
are more commonly first noted in
teenage or early adult life.

Another pattern of idiopathic
calcinosis cutis is also found in
children, and may be present at birth.
There is usually a single hard nodule
on the face (a), usually covered by
hyperkeratotic epidermis; this pattern
is sometimes known as a subepidermal
calcified nodule.

In both patterns there are roughly
spherical nodules of calcium in the
dermis, surrounded by a fibrous tissue
response (b) with occasional histiocytes
and giant cells, but rarely the florid
granulomatous response seen around
urate crystals in gout (see Fig. 11.8).

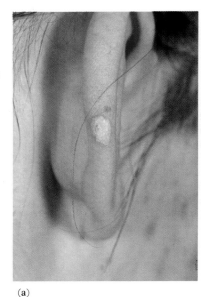

(a)

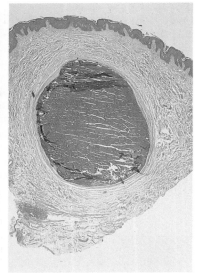

(b)

16. Basal cell carcinoma

Introduction

Basal cell carcinoma (BCC) occurs on hair-bearing skin and increases in incidence with age. BCC is common over the age of 50 in both sexes, especially on light-exposed areas such as the central part of the face and forehead. It is uncommon on the limbs. Predisposing factors include UV and ionising radiation, and exposure to inorganic arsenic; multiple lesions are not uncommon and may be due to genetic predisposition.

The characteristic cell type of this tumour has a large dark-staining nucleus and a peripheral rim of scanty, pale-staining cytoplasm with an indistinct cell membrane. The cells are usually tightly packed together, but their arrangement and disposition with regard to one another is very variable.

There are several histological patterns of basal cell carcinoma, the definition of which may indicate the likely clinical behaviour of a lesion following excision. The five main patterns are nodular BCC (and cystic variant), morphoeic BCC, superficial multifocal BCC, and keratotic BCC. Excess melanin deposition may occur in the basal cells to produce a pigmented appearance (pigmented BCC). A characteristic feature of the histology of all types of basal cell carcinoma is nests of tumour cells where the peripheral cells are arranged in a regular row, a feature known as palisading (Fig. 16.1(c)). Palisading may be difficult to find in the morphoeic pattern.

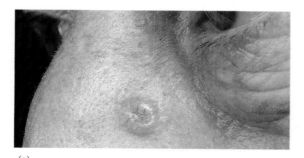

(a)

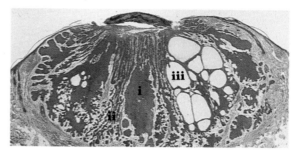

(b)

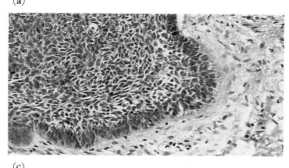

(c)

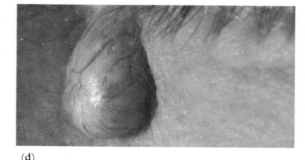

(d)

Fig. 16.1(a)–(d). Nodular basal cell carcinoma

This is the commonest type; it presents as a firm raised papule or nodule with a translucent 'pearly' edge, over which run prominent telangiectatic vessels, usually radially. The apex of the nodule eventually develops a central depression and ulceration; deep and lateral extension of the tumour, with invasive destruction of adjacent and underlying tissues, produces enlarging ulceration, the so-called 'rodent ulcer'.

In (a), note the typical location, the shiny, pearly colour of the edge, the prominent telangiectatic vessels, and the small ulcer at the peak. The characteristic pearly appearance is due to the undermining of the thinned normal epidermis by white tumour, as shown in (b); the telangiectatic vessels

are dilated upper dermal capillaries 'trapped' between the thin covering epidermis and the undermining tumour mass. The tumour has ulcerated through the thin epidermis at the apex of the dome-shaped nodule; a scab sits in the ulcer crater. This example shows a mixed histological pattern of solid lobular (i), trabecular (ii) and cystic (iii) areas. The high-power photomicrograph (c) shows the palisading pattern seen at the periphery of the tumour lobules; this is the most characteristic histological feature of basal cell carcinomas; (d) shows a typical cystic basal cell carcinoma, in which the tumour is almost entirely composed of the histological pattern (iii) in (b). Note also in (d) the prominent telangiectasia due to prominent vessels beneath the thinned stretched epidermis.

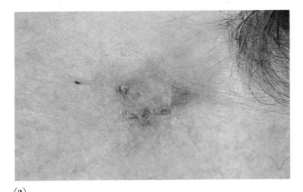

(a)

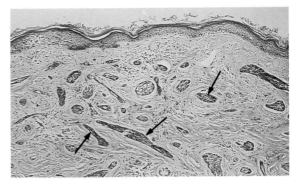

(b)

Fig. 16.2(a), (b) & (c). Morphoeic basal cell carcinoma

Clinically, this pattern of basal cell carcinoma appears as a white-yellow thickened plaque or area of sunken atrophic skin which may have indistinct edges and be ulcerated (a), often in several sites within the plaque. The tumour may extend for some distance beyond the visible borders. They usually occur on the face, and if present in nasolabial fold or inner canthus, their removal is a major surgical problem.

The neoplastic basal cells are present in small compressed clumps and irregular columns (arrows) embedded in dense fibrous stroma in the dermis, hence the impression of thickening (b). In this variant, peripheral palisading is often scanty and may be absent, particularly where the fibrous stroma is substantial. Often the continuity between epidermis and the tumour cells in the dermis is not apparent, as here. The lesion is often depressed below the surface of the rest of the skin.

A variant which shows similar excessive fibrous reaction in the dermis is the so-called 'fibro-epithelioma of Pinkus'. This differs histologically from morphoeic basal

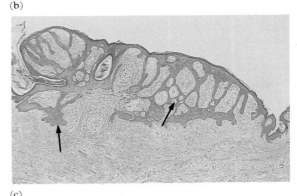

(c)

cell carcinoma in that the tumour cells form an intricate pattern of narrow interconnecting strands (arrows in (c)); clinically, the two are quite distinct, fibro-epithelioma usually appearing as a raised papule, often on the trunk.

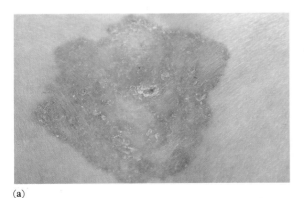

(a)

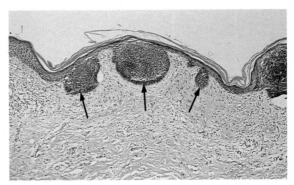

(b)

Fig. 16.3(a) & (b). Superficial basal cell carcinoma

This usually presents as a flat, red plaque with an irregular scalloped edge which often has a distinct translucent raised rim. Sometimes the centre is scaly and atrophic as in this example (a). They are commonest on the trunk and face, and may be confused clinically with intra-epidermal carcinoma. Multiple lesions may be associated with previous exposure to inorganic arsenic or irradiation.

Histologically, this lesion shows small buds or irregular downgrowths of palisaded basal cells extending into the upper dermis from the lower border of the epidermis. Such downgrowths are frequently multiple (arrowed in (b)), hence the commonly used adjective 'multicentric' applied to this lesion. There is usually a proliferation of cellular fibrous tissue in the upper dermis around the basal cell clumps, together with a variable chronic inflammatory cell infiltrate.

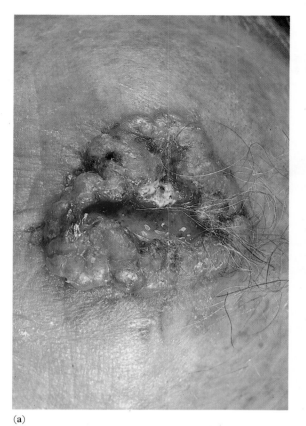

(a)

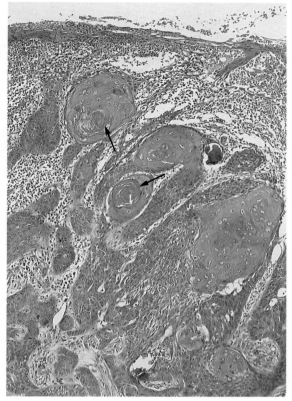

(b)

Fig. 16.4(a) & (b). Keratotic basal cell carcinoma

These lesions can look most unlike the previous descriptions and the diagnosis may only be made histologically. They have a central crust of keratin which may be removed to reveal a bleeding ulcer, and there is sometimes atrophy and telangiectasia. They are most frequent on the scalp (a) and legs.

The histological characteristic of this lesion is the presence of keratin aggregates (inaccurately called 'horn cysts') within the islands of basal cell carcinomas, usually in

the form of spherical masses surrounded by parakeratotic flattened cells (arrows in (b)). Keratohyaline granules are absent. The pattern may be confused histologically with trichoepithelioma although they are clinically distinct (see Fig. 20.5) and the presence of keratin may lead to an erroneous diagnosis of mixed basal and squamous carcinoma (basosquamous carcinoma or metatypical basal carcinoma), an entity which is currently considered doubtful.

Fig. 16.5. Pigmented basal cell carcinoma

The histological features are usually those of a nodular or possibly superficial BCC, but there is brown-black melanin in neoplastic basal cells. Clinical distinction from melanoma maybe difficult.

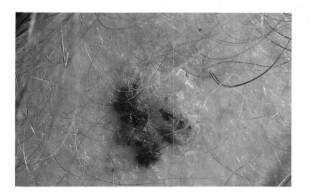

17. Benign dyskeratoses and squamous keratoses

Introduction

Excessive or abnormal keratin production is a frequent secondary feature of many disorders of different aetiologies and pathogeneses illustrated in other chapters in this book, e.g. viral wart. The excess keratin may be either orthokeratotic or parakeratotic (see Fig. 4.14), or a mixture of both. In this chapter we deal with a number of skin lesions, characterized by generalized or localized hyperkeratosis, which do not fit comfortably into other chapters, or are unclassifiable because their pathogenesis is poorly understood. The terms 'dyskeratoses' and 'benign squamous keratoses' are sometimes used to describe such conditions.

Generalized excessive keratin production is the characteristic feature of the group of conditions referred to clinically as the *ichthyoses*, in which the thick surface keratin layer is not usually associated with acanthotic thickening of the epidermis. In almost all the other dyskeratoses and squamous keratoses the epidermal layer is abnormally thick, and may be qualitatively abnormal too; for example, there may be acantholysis, as in Darier's disease and warty dyskeratoma.

Many benign squamous keratoses are surgically removed very late in their natural history, by which time they may be extremely hyperkeratotic and show the histological effects of long-standing trauma with secondary inflammatory changes. At this stage they may show no specific features which would allow the nature of the underlying epidermal abnormality to be identified with certainty. Sometimes the hyperkeratosis is very marked and localized, producing a hard protruberance of compacted keratin called a cutaneous horn (Fig. 17.7). It is important to identify the epidermal abnormality at the base of a cutaneous horn since there may be underlying epidermal dysplasia such as solar keratosis or intra-epidermal carcinoma, although cutaneous horns also arise on viral warts, epidermal naevus and seborrhoeic keratosis.

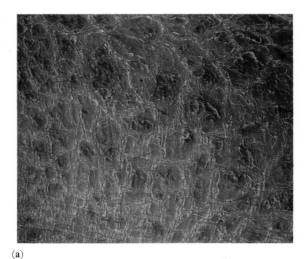

(a)

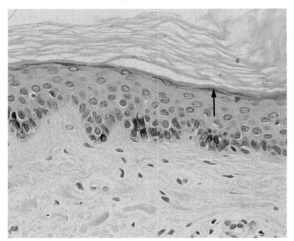

(b)

Fig. 17.1 (a) & (b) Ichthyosis

Ichthyosis is a general term used to describe a fish-like scaliness of the skin. Usually ichthyosis is inherited, although it can develop in patients with lymphoma and other internal malignancies as an acquired condition. The pattern of inheritance varies according to the type of ichthyosis (see Table 17.1), and in some types evidence of an underlying biochemical disorder is emerging; in sex-linked recessive ichthyosis there is an absence of, or greatly reduced, steroid sulphatase activity in the epidermal cells, white blood cells, and probably other cells; this is thought to

lead to increased cell cohesion in the granular and prickle cell layers, thus retarding the shedding of keratin at the skin surface.

Figure 17.1(a) shows the typical clinical appearance of ichthyosis; note the excessive scaliness; histologically there is hyperkeratosis, which is a constant feature of all ichthyotic lesions, but there are variations in the changes seen in the epidermal layers according to type. For example, the granular layer is insignificant or absent in the vulgaris pattern, but present in sex-linked recessive ichthyosis (arrowed in (b)).

Table 17.1   Patterns of ichthyosis

Type	Inheritance	Scale pattern	Other features
Ichthyosis vulgaris	Autosomal dominant	Fine, white	Granular layer absent; improves with age.
Sex-linked recessive	Sex-lined recessive	Coarse, dark	Granular layer present; no improvement with age.
Ichthyosiform erythroderma	Autosomal recessive	Large, verrucous	Associated erythroderma, ectropion.
Bullous ichthyosiform erythroderma	Autosomal dominant	Thick, brown verrucous	Bullous in early childhood, hyperkeratosis later.

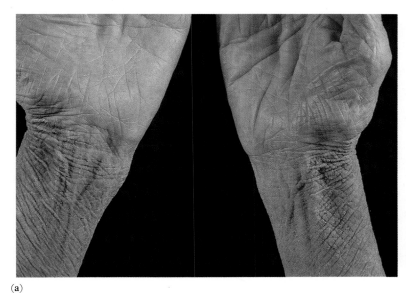

(a)

Fig. 17.2 (a) & (b) Acanthosis nigricans
The name is misleading because acanthosis is often not particularly prominent and certainly not enough to account for the thickened warty appearance which is the result of hyperkeratosis and epidermal folding. Despite this the skin is often smooth and velvety; the dirty brown colour is also a result of hyperkeratosis rather than melanin (a). Lesions are mild and confined to flexures when acanthosis nigricans is due to obesity, when it is probably a local response to friction. It may affect the whole skin with thickened palms and oral hyperkeratosis when it is associated with adenocarcinoma. Histologically, there is marked but irregular hyperkeratosis and prominent papillomatosis (b). There is rarely excessive melanin pigmentation in the lesion.

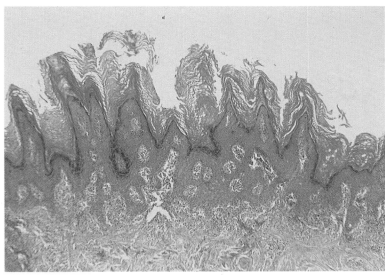

(b)

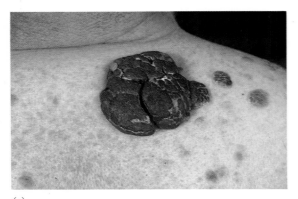

(a)

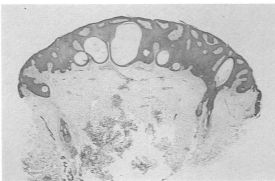

(b)

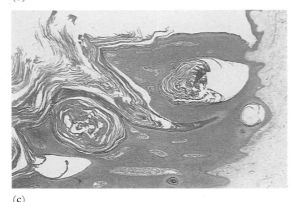

(c)

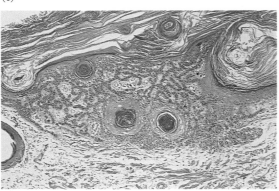

(d)

Fig. 17.3 (a)–(d) Seborrhoeic keratosis

This lesion is extremely common, increasing in number with age, so that in the elderly they are usually multiple; they are uncommon below the age of 35. Clinically, they appear as raised brown or grey lesions with a 'greasy' appearance and feel, hence their name. Characteristically, they have a warty surface with well-defined markings and a sharply outlined raised edge, giving a 'stuck-on' appearance (a).

Histologically, the common feature of these lesions is the proliferation within the epidermis of basal cells, producing a raised lesion capped with a variable amount of surface hyperkeratosis. A number of different patterns of the lesion exists. The most common pattern is illustrated in Figure 17.3(b); there is marked acanthosis in which the thickened epidermis is largely composed of tightly packed small dark-staining basal cells. Almost invariably present are roughly spherical masses of keratin surrounded by a narrow rim of epidermal cells showing some squamous differentiation. Occasionally, this squamous change is so marked that it dominates the histological picture and the basal cell component appears minor; this type is usually associated with very thick surface hyperkeratosis, producing a dirty, gray, warty surface appearance. The extensive squamous change is thought to be result of chronic irritation and repeated trauma; see Figure 17.3(c).

Less common variants include the adenoid or trabecular pattern (d) and the clonal or 'basal nest' pattern.

All patterns may show excessive melanin pigmentation.

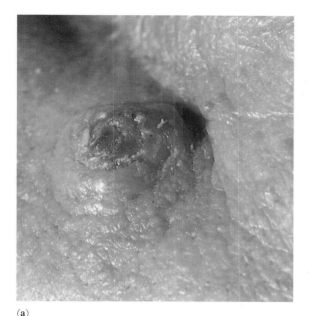

(a)

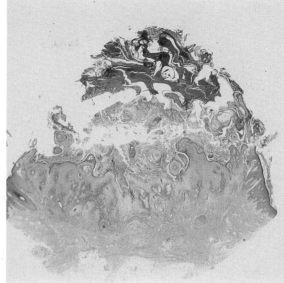

(b)

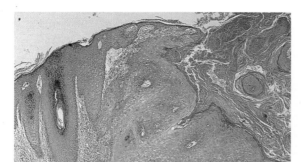

(c)

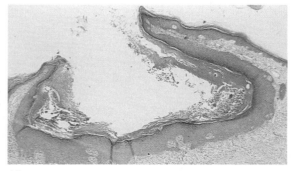

(d)

Fig. 17.4 (a)–(d) Keratoacanthoma

The most striking feature of keratoacanthoma is its rapid growth: maximum size is usually attained in 6–8 weeks, following which there is equally rapid regression. The lesion begins as a red papule, and evolves into a 2–3 cm domed nodule with a translucent, often telangiectatic, raised edge and a central keratin plug(a). The edges gradually shrink but remain raised with a depressed flat centre, eventually leaving a pitted scar. The face is a common site but they can occur anywhere. If there is doubt about the diagnosis it is best to excise the whole lesion but where this is inappropiate, a large incisional biopsy should include the edge and some normal skin. Curettte biopsies are much less satisfactory but are often sent to the laboratory following therapeutic curettage of a clinically definite keratoacanthoma.

The histological appearance of keratoacanthoma varies according to the stage of development reached at the time of excision. When biopsied at the peak of its activity, when the central keratinous plug is prominent, the histological features are fairly characteristic. At low magnification, the lesion is a roughly rounded invagination of thickened epidermis with a central crater filled with irregular masses of keratin (b). The rim of the crater is formed by a lip of normal epidermis stretched thin over the undermining mass

of hyperplastic epidermis (c). This distinct lip is a useful distinguishing feature from squamous carcinoma (c). The lower border of a keratoacanthoma is usually irregular, and the demarcation between dermis and epidermis is often unclear, mimicking malignant invasion. At high magnification the hyperplastic cells show cytoplasmic and nuclear atypia, with increase in mitotic activity, another factor leading to confusion with squamous carcinoma. However, within keratoacanthoma will usually be found some areas in which the epidermal cells will be swollen and palely eosinophilic with a rather homogeneous glassy appearance, suggesting virus-infected cells.

In early lesions, the epidermal proliferation is more pronounced and the central keratin plug is smaller. At this actively proliferating stage a keratoacanthoma may be histologically indistinguishable from squamous carcinoma, particularly in an incision biopsy. A complete excision biopsy is essential.

An old, incompletely resolved keratoacanthoma may cause diagnostic difficulty, clinically and histologically. With the passage of time the active epidermal proliferation abates, and the lesion flattens as the central depression becomes larger and shallower, the plug of keratin is extruded and eroded away, and is not replaced as the activity of the epidermis dies down (d).

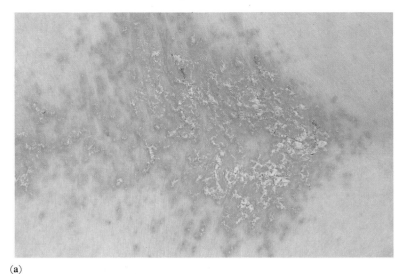

(a)

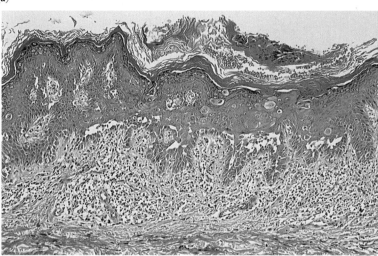

(b)

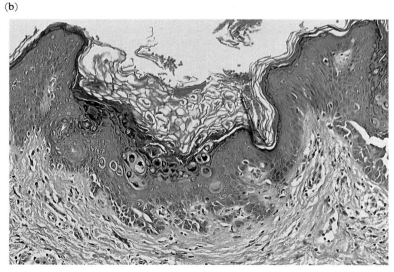

(c)

Fig. 17.5(a), (b) & (c) Darier's disease

This is dominantly inherited and usually presents in adolescence as sheets of hard keratotic papules, usually on the scalp and flexures(a). There is often secondary bacterial infection. Nail keratin is brittle and breaks easily, leaving v-shaped notches, and there are tiny papules and pits on the palms and soles. Although suprabasal acantholysis occurs, this almost never gives rise to a blistering lesion, despite the formation of focal clefts in the epidermis just above the basal layer (b). The acantholysis is associated with dyskeratosis, and the epidermis above the focus of acantholyic clefting is occupied by dyskeratotic cells, including the characteristic 'corps ronds'; see Figure 4.6(b). The acantholytic dyskeratotic keratinocytes give rise to a localized column of parakeratosis, usually with a surrounding zone of orthokeratotic hyperkeratosis. Lesions are focal but multiple (c).

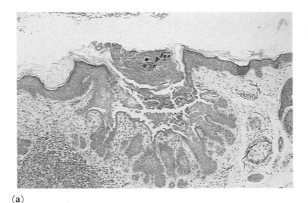

(a)

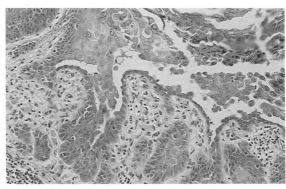

(b)

Fig. 17.6(a) & (b) Warty dyskeratoma

This lesion occurs most commonly on the face or neck and occasionally in the scalp. It is usually a solitary, raised, dome-shaped papule with a central pit or umbilication from which keratin may protrude.

Histologically, warty dyskeratoma is characterized by the presence of extensive acantholysis of the squamous epidermis lining a spherical pit which is filled with keratin. At low magnification (a) the lower border of the lesion

appears clearly defined and rounded, but at high magnification (b) it can be seen to have a more or less regularly convoluted appearance due to finger-like villi of dermal papillary tissue intruding into the lumen of the depression (a); these villi are often covered only by a thin layer of basal cells, the other cells having been shed (as a result of acantholysis) into the lumen of the pit where they can be seen as acantholytic dyskeratotic cells intermingling with the keratin (b).

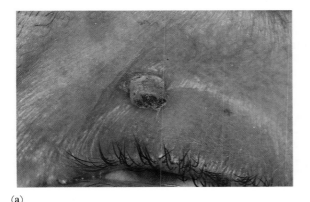

(a)

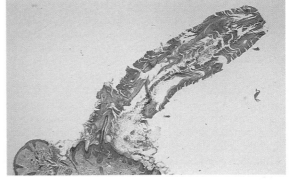

(b)

Fig. 17.7(a) & (b) Cutaneous horn

Cutaneous horns occur most commonly in the elderly. They are hard, protruding, keratinous lumps (as their name suggests) usually with normal-appearing skin immediately adjacent to their base (a). Redness or scaling of the base implies trauma or epidermal dysplasia.

Micrograph (b) shows a cutaneous horn based on an old, now inactive, viral wart. A heavy lymphocytic infiltrate in the underlying dermis is a frequent finding, irrespective of the nature of the causative lesion and is probably the result of repeated episodes of trauma.

18. Actinic keratosis, carcinoma in situ, and squamous cell carcinoma

Introduction

In normal epidermis, basal cells proliferate and produce keratinocytes of the prickle cell and granular cell layers. This normal structural gradient of the epidermis may alter under various pathological stimuli; for example, an increase in the number of basal cells will occur as a response to cell loss through inflammation or trauma. This type of alteration of growth will revert to normal if the stimulus causing it is removed. The term *hyperplasia* is applied to this reversible adaptive increase in the proliferative rate of the epidermis, and common causes in the skin include viral infection of keratinocytes (see Figs. 10.2, 10.5, 10.6) and repeated trauma or irritation. Hyperplastic proliferation of epidermis produces thick prickle and granular cell layers (acanthosis and hypergranulosis; see Figs. 4.2 and 4.13a) and an increase in the overlying keratin layer(hyperkeratosis; see Fig. 4.14). Hyperplasia is mentioned here to contrast it with the situation where increased cell proliferation persists even after the stimulus which originally caused it has been eliminated; this is called *neoplasia*, and the proliferating cells usually show cytological abnormalities (cellular atypia or dysplasia), which is not usually a prominent feature of hyperplastic overgrowth.

In neoplastic proliferations of the keratinocytes of the epidermis, two basic divisions are made:
1. The abnormal cells are confined by the basement membrane (carcinoma in situ);
2. The abnormal cells grow into the dermis and other structures (invasive carcinoma). In epidermal neoplasia, cytological atypia, recognised by large abnormal nuclei, increased numbers of cells in mitosis, and abnormal mitoses, is associated with complete loss of the normal pattern of cell maturation.

An intermediate state of abnormal epidermal cell growth, between hyperplasia and neoplasia, exists in the skin and many other epithelia in the body; this is called *dysplasia*, because cellular atypia is its most significant feature. There is histological evidence of abnormal proliferation with increase in mitoses, failure of normal maturation, and cells which cytologically resemble those seen in carcinoma. There is, however, only a partial loss of maturation; polarity of the epidermis, although disturbed, is not lost completely. The condition falls short of carcinoma in situ and is not a simple hyperplasia because of the abnormal cytology of cells. This type of abnormal epidermal growth is seen in actinic keratosis. It must be emphasised that the distinction between carcinoma in situ and dysplasia is a histological one and the division implies a predictive statement on the further behaviour of a lesion. An actinic keratosis is a benign dysplastic condition and will not metastasize, although an invasive carcinoma may develop in a pre-existing actinic keratosis. A carcinoma in situ in skin is a malignant neoplasm because the cells have the potential to invade.

The histological changes from mild dysplasia through severe dyplasia to carcinoma in situ form a continuum with the same types of abnormalities present in increasing degrees. These lesions are associated with an increased risk of the local development of invasive squamous carcinoma. In actinic keratosis this is small and is higher for established carcinoma in situ.

It is important to distinguish the processes of epidermal regeneration and hyperplasia from neoplasia. In some examples of regenerative hyperplasia there may be many of the cytological features of neoplastic cells, including pleomorphism, hyperchromatism, and mitotic activity. Usually there are other features which suggest that atypia of squamous epithelium is secondary to an initiating event. If the atypical epithelium is present only in areas of acute inflammation or overlies a zone of granulation tissue then this suggests that the cellular atypia is regenerative and secondary to inflammation. When atypia is the sole abnormality and without any recognizable cause, neoplasia should be suspected. Occasionally regenerative or viral-induced hyperplasia may simulate invasive carcinoma, hence the term pseudocarcinomatous hyperplasia. While this may be of use to the histologist as a reminder to consider other causes of atypical hyperplasia, it is a confusing term and should not appear in pathological descriptions. An example of a localized epidermal hyperplasia which may be difficult to distinguish from invasive squamous carcinoma, both clinically and histologically, is keratoacanthoma which is discussed and illustrated in Fig. 17.4.

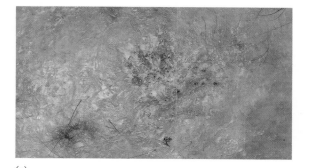

(a)

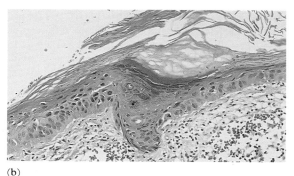

(b)

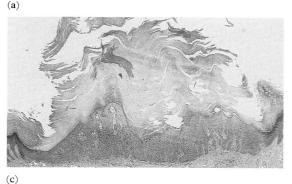

(c)

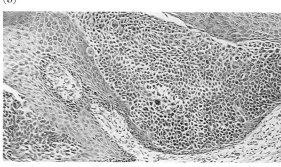

(d)

Fig. 18.1 (a)–(d) Actinic (solar) keratosis
This is a form of epidermal dysplasia; actinic keratoses are frequently multiple and found in association with mottled pigmentation and the yellowish smooth dermal plaques characteristic of actinic or solar elastosis. They are most numerous on the face, scalp, forearms and backs of the hands. The lesions are approximately 0.5–1 cm in size and are characterized by a rough, hard, keratotic irregular surface. The keratin is often a dirty brown colour and firmly stuck onto the skin; its removal results in bleeding. There may be telangectasia visible through the adjacent, often thinned, epidermis, giving the lesion a reddish colour and an ill-defined edge and sometimes they may appear depressed because of epidermal atrophy combined with loss of collagen (a). Keratoses due to ionizing radiation and arsenic have similar morphology; arsenical keratoses are common on palms and soles.

The main histological features common to all actinic keratoses are epidermal keratinocytes with enlarged nuclei which are irregular in size and shape (nuclear pleomorphism). The nuclei stain more darkly than normal with haematoxylin (hyperchromatism), and there may be increased numbers of mitoses in all layers of the epidermis. Keratinization is abnormal with premature keratinization of isolated cells at various depths in the epidermis (dyskeratosis; see Fig. 4.6). Surface keratinization is abnormal with parakeratosis which may be of great thickness, occasionally forming a cutaneous horn (see Fig. 17.7).

The architecture of the epidermis is altered. Pleomorphic cells with hyperchromatic nuclei replace much of the lower part of the epithelium and may be seen occasionally near the surface. Polarity of the epidermis is roughly preserved, with proliferation occurring in the lower portion and maturation near the surface. When the pleomorphic changes occupy the whole thickness of the epidermis and there is no maturation near the surface the lesion is a carcinoma in situ (see Fig. 18.2).

Histopathologists recognize a number of patterns of actinic keratosis, based on variations in histological appearance: classical, atrophic, hyperplastic, acantholytic and 'Bowenoid' patterns of actinic keratosis.

In Figure 18.1(b), an example of an *atrophic actinic keratosis*, there is loss of rete ridges and the epithelium is reduced to 5 or 6 cells in thickness. Careful inspection of the nuclear detail reveals the diagnostic pleomorphism and disturbance of keratinization. Note that there is surface parakeratosis and a non-specific chronic inflammatory infiltrate in the upper dermis.

In *hypertrophic actinic keratosis* (c) there is thickening of the epidermis which is occasionally of papillary configuration. The features of epithelial dysplasia are present. This type of lesion is sometimes confused with seborrhoeic keratosis on low power examination. It is important to look at the regularity of nuclei of all lesions with the morphology of a seborrhoeic keratosis to avoid this error.

In *Bowenoid actinic keratosis* (d) the lower part of the epidermis is replaced by discontinuous nests of atypical dysplastic cells. Occasional nuclei in these nests are greatly enlarged, up to 6 times the size of other cells. It is important to examine carefully all of the tissue in such lesions since deeper levels will often show that there is full thickness replacement of the epidermis by dysplastic keratinocytes further in the tissue block, indicating that the lesion is really a carcinoma in situ in which the malignant cells have infiltrated the lower layers of surrounding epidermis by lateral spread. A sharp discontinuity between the atypical and the superficial normal mature epithelium is a clue to this phenomenon. At first sight these lesions may resemble a clonal seborrhoeic keratosis, and careful scrutiny at high magnification to identify atypical cells is essential.

In *acantholytic actinic keratosis* there are foci of acantholysis with small cleft-like spaces developing in the lower and mid-portions of the epithelium within the atypical areas.

Squamous carcinoma in situ (intra-epidermal carcinoma)

Carcinoma in situ is carcinoma confined within epidermis by the basement membrane. Erythroplasia of Queyrat and Bowen's disease are eponyms which should no longer be used. In the vulval skin, a nomenclature has been adopted by gynaecological pathologists to term atypical proliferation of the epidermis as Vulval In situ Neoplasia or VIN. VIN 1 and 2 correspond to mild and moderate dysplasia, while VIN 3 corresponds to in situ carcinoma.

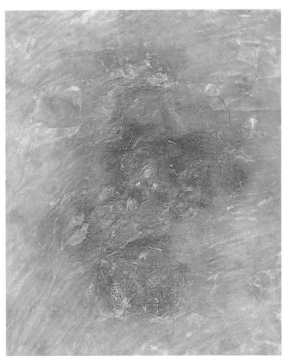

(a)

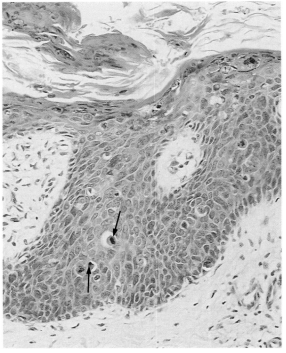

(b)

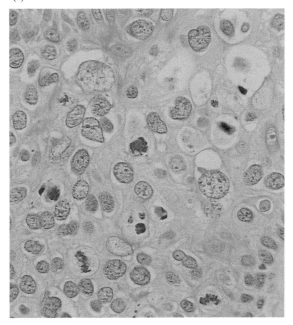

(c)

Fig. 18.2 (a), (b) & (c) Intra-epidermal carcinoma (IEC)

In situ epidermal carcinoma (IEC) appears as red-brown, often flat or slightly raised plaques with a scaly, sometimes eroded, surface and a fairly well-defined edge (a). Lesions are frequent on the trunk and limbs, usually in the over 50s. Thickness is determined both by the amount of accumulated scale and by the thickness of the proliferating zone of the epidermis: in general the thicker it is, the likelier that there is invasion of the dermis. Multiple lesions are frequently a legacy of inorganic arsenic toxicity (usually given as a 'tonic' in childhood). Rather like psoriasis (which lesions may resemble), the appearance is modified in flexural areas to a smooth glazed, often eroded, plaque which may also resemble extra-mammary Paget's disease. Occasionally the lesions are hyperkeratotic.

Histologically, there is acanthosis, hyperkeratosis and parakeratosis. The epidermal cells are replaced by keratinocytes which show nuclear pleomorphism and hyperchromatism. Mitotic figures are seen above the basal layer, and disturbed keratinization is manifest as dyskeratotic cells (arrow in (b)). The fine cytological features are seen at high magnification in a thin resin section (c). Beneath the lesion, actinic degeneration of collagen is a frequent occurrence in those lesions developing in sun exposed skin. In contrast to actinic keratosis, the atypical changes affect the full thickness of the epidermis.

Invasive squamous carcinoma

Invasive squamous carcinoma of the skin can arise *de novo* but commonly arises in an area of previous epidermal dysplasia. However, the probability of individual actinic keratoses becoming malignant is very low— a recent estimate is 0.25% — and dysplasia invisible to the naked eye is very common as evidenced by the large areas revealed by treatment of actinic keratoses with topical 5 fluoruracil. The risk for in situ carcinoma is much greater. It may also occur in association with chronic inflammatory conditions of the skin such as the margin of an ulcer, or in scars due to radiation dermatitis or burns.

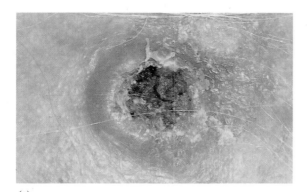

(a)

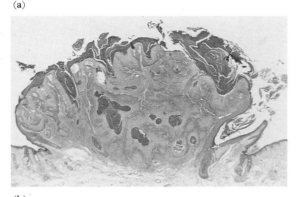

(b)

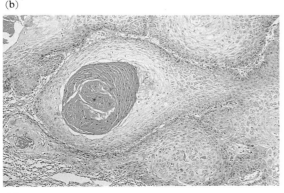

(c)

Fig. 18.3 (a), (b) & (c) Invasive squamous carcinoma

Clinically, squamous carcinomas are usually fairly rapidly growing lesions which therefore present as nodules of densely packed proliferating keratinocytes. There is a raised, rather translucent, solid-feeling edge surrounded by erythema and with a central ulcer (a). Less well-differentiated lesions may produce so much local destruction that they simply appear as bleeding, indurated ulcers filled with crust and keratin; there is usually an indistinct oedematous edge. The lesion may be fixed to adjacent structures. Common sites include face, scalp, lower lip, and the backs of forearms and hands.

Histologically, squamous cell carcinoma of the skin may exhibit varying degrees of differentiation and may be termed *well, moderately* or *poorly differentiated* according to the degree of maturation seen in the tumour, particularly the extent of keratin formation and the preservation of prickle cell characteristics.

In a *well-differentiated squamous carcinoma*, as shown in this example from the pinna (b) there may be hyperkeratosis, parakeratotis, or crusting ulceration over an area of proliferating keratinocytes. Cytologically, the cells exhibit features of atypia with pleormorphism, nuclear hyperchromatism, and increase in mitoses. There is maturation to a flattened keratinized cell; however, this may be premature and be represented as isolated dyskeratoses. The main feature of this lesion is invasion of the dermis by the proliferating cells. In many cases, these invading cells form islands of tumour in the dermis with a central zone of pink-staining keratinization (keratin 'pearl') (c). Lesions which may be confused with a well-differentiated squamous cell carcinoma include keratoacanthoma, and areas of reactive epidermal hyperplasia such as seen in the edge of an ulcerated area.

Verrucous carcinoma of the skin is commonly seen in the vulva. In this type of lesion there is a predominantly exophytic and papillary growth pattern of the epidermis with only moderate atypia of keratinocytes. There is commonly extensive hyperkeratosis. This lesion is associated with a low incidence of metastasis and tends to recur locally, behaving as a low grade carcinoma. Histologically, the difficulty with these lesions is that they show little of the cytological characteristics of malignancy, and can be confused with benign hyperplastic lesions. Clinically too, they can be confused with vulval condylomas.

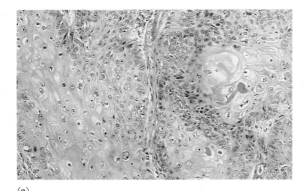

(a)

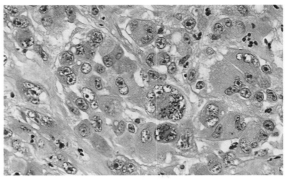

(b)

Fig. 18.4(a) & (b) Poorly differentiated squamous carcinoma

In a *poorly differentiated squamous carcinoma* (a), there is less maturation to a keratinocyte and a marked degree of pleomorphism with frequent mitoses. Cells in these lesions have a high nuclear to cytoplasmic ratio, and the cytoplasm stains less pink than a normal keratinocyte. Evidence of squamous origin is revealed by intercellular junctions seen as 'prickles' between adjacent cells at a high magnification.

As in the in-situ lesion, acantholysis may occur between the tumour cells to produce a 'pseudoglandular' pattern. Micrograph (b) shows a tumour which is so poorly differentiated that its origin from epidermal keratinocytes is not apparent on H & E stain, and it resembles a pleomorphic malignant melanoma. In such difficult cases, electron microscopy and immunocytochemical methods may be required to identify the tumour type (see below).

At the worst end of the spectrum are undifferentiated lesions which may be pleomorphic or spindle cell in pattern and be confused with sarcoma, or melanoma (see Fig. 18.4(b)). Immunocytochemistry and electron microscopy are of use in the differential diagnosis of this type of lesion. True spindle cell squamous carcinomas will show persisting desmosomal cell junctions and cytoplasmic tonofibrils on electron microscopy, no matter how poorly differentiated the tumour. Poorly differentiated melanoma can be identified by the presence in the cytoplasm of melanosomes and premelanosomes (see Fig. 3.6), even if the tumour is so undifferentiated that it is not producing demonstrable melanin. Spindle cell sarcomas show neither premelanosomes nor desmosomal cell junctions, and their content of cytoplasmic organelles can sometimes be used to identify their cell of origin.

Immunocytochemical identification of fairly specific cell markers, although in its infancy, can be used to identify the cell of origin of poorly differentiated tumours. In the case of spindle cell tumours in skin, the reactions with a panel of two markers can usually help to identify the nature of the tumour. Melanoma expresses S100 protein but not cytokeratin. Squamous carcinoma expresses cytokeratin but not S100 protein.

19. Melanocytic lesions

Introduction

Normal melanocytes are discussed and illustrated in detail in Chapter 3 (see Figs. 3.4, 3.5, and 3.6).

Physiological increase in the rate of melanin production leads to freckles (ephelides) which appear in childhood on exposed sites; they have a uniform pale-brown colour and darken after exposure to sunlight. This distinguishes them from lentigo which is also a pigmented macule.

In an ephelis the epidermal cells are histologically normal; the macular pigmented lesion is recognizable as a circumscribed zone of basal cells containing excess melanin. Melanocytes are present in normal numbers in the basal layer. While this type of lesion is not usually excised, its histological recognition is important to avoid confusion with other pigmented lesions.

There are two main groups of lesions of melanocytes. The commonest by far is benign overgrowth of melanocytes, termed *melanocytic naevi*. These lesions are common, resulting in the various types of clinically and pathologically identifiable naevi, often regarded as hamartomatous.

Secondly, there are pre-malignant and malignant proliferations of melanocytes, termed *dysplastic or atypical naevi* and *malignant melanoma* respectively.

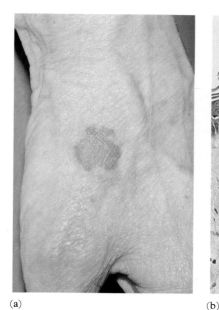

(a)

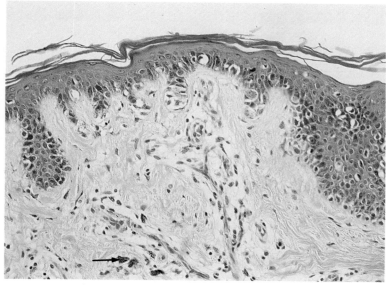

(b)

Fig. 19.1(a) & (b) Benign lentigo

Clinically, these are distinguished from freckles because they can occur at any age and at any site, tend to be darker brown, and sun exposure does not change their colour. In childhood they may be associated with the Peutz-Jegher syndrome.

Histologically, there is increase in basal melanocyte numbers in the basal layer of the epidermis, and there is mild to moderate acanthosis of the epidermis with slight bulbous swellings at the tips of rete ridges. Melanin pigment may be present at all levels in the epidermis and melanin-containing macrophages are present in the upper dermis (arrow in (b)), occasionally associated with a mild lymphocytic infiltrate.

In the elderly, lentigos gradually develop as pale brown macules on exposed sites such as the face and forearms (liver spots, senile lentigo) (a). Histologically, this group shows budding and downgrowth of the basal layer of the epidermis often in an irregular pattern, in contrast to lentigo simplex which tends to be regular. Melanin pigment is present mainly at the lower ends of the basal layer downgrowths and melanocytes are slightly increased in the basal layer (b).

Melanocytic naevi

A melanocytic naevus is a localized overgrowth of melanocytes. Clinically and histologically they can be divided into several types, depending on appearance and structure:

1. Junctional naevus;
2. Compound naevus;
3. Intradermal naevus;
4. Blue naevus;
5. Spitz naevus (juvenile melanoma).

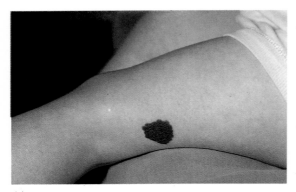

(a)

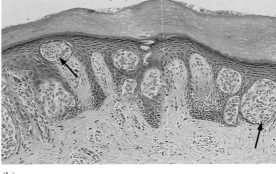

(b)

Fig. 19.2(a) & (b) Junctional naevus.

Junctional naevi are usually uniformly dark-brown macules with a smooth, well-defined edge. They appear mostly between childhood and adolescence; their sudden appearance in adulthood is unusual and should be regarded with suspicion.

The junctional naevus is characterized by proliferation of melanocytes in the basal layer of the epidermis only. The melanocytes form rounded balls of cells which appear to bulge down into the upper dermis. However, all of these

cells are intra-epidermal, being contained within epidermal basal lamina, and are termed junctional nests. When this pattern of proliferation occupies the majority of the naevus it is termed an active junctional naevus, and must be distinguished from atypical melanocytic proliferation.

Histologically, rounded nests of melanocytes (arrows in (b)) are present in the basal layer of the epidermis pushing down into the upper dermis. There is no upward growth of melanocytes, and no dermal melanocyte component (b). A junctional naevus may surround a hair follicle.

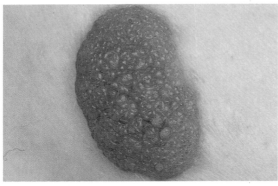

(a)

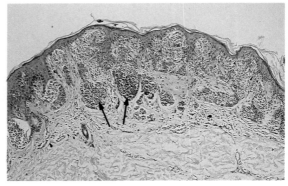

(b)

Fig. 19.3(a) & (b) Compound naevus.

Compound naevi are raised, often with an irregular, folded, papilliferous surface, but retain uniformity of colour and outline(a). Stippling of pigment does occur, but greater variegation than this is not a feature and could suggest malignancy. Hair growth within the lesion is common. These lesions tend to occur later than junctional naevi, i.e. from the 2nd to the 4th decade.

In a compound naevus, naevus cells are seen both in

the epidermis, forming junctional nests as in the junctional naevus, but also in the dermis, where rounded cell nests are separated by dermal collagen (arrows). It is postulated that junctional nests become detached from the basal layer with re-growth of basal lamina above the nests and overgrowth of dermal connective tissue. Histologically, the junctional component and rounded dermal nests of melanocytes are well shown in (b).

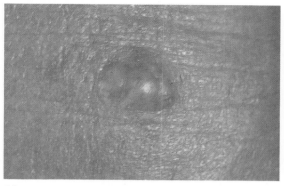

(a)

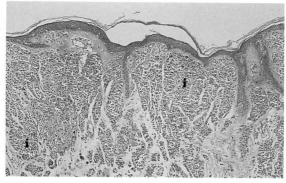

(b)

Fig. 19.4(a) & (b) Intradermal naevi

Intradermal naevi are also raised, usually being smooth, shiny-surfaced, domed papules, flesh-coloured or slightly stippled with brown (a). They usually develop in adults and are uncommon under the age of 20.

Histologically, they show no evidence of a junctional component and are composed of nests of melanocytes **(i)** within the dermis. They produce little melanin, hence their clinical appearance. In this type of naevus and in the deeper parts of the compound naevus there may be heavy collagenization, with spindle cell areas of naevus cells resembling nerve sheath Schwann cells. This 'neuroid' pattern is frequently seen in older lesions and may represent

maturation of the naevus with ageing. A common feature of intradermal components is occasional multinucleate melanocytes forming giant cells. This is not evidence of cellular atypia and is a feature of benign lesions. A histological curio is the occurrence of some melanocytes which have a large extremely vacuolated appearance and a dense, stained, rounded and often central nucleus. When such cells form the main component of a naevus it is termed a *balloon cell naevus*.

Congenital melanocytic naevi are present at birth and may be of large size. Giant congenital naevi carry the risk of malignant change.

Fig. 19.5 Halo naevus

Pigmented naevi which develop depigmentation or hypopigmentation of the peripheral normal skin are called halo naevi. This usually occurs on the trunk during the 2nd to 3rd decades. The halo is uniformly pale and symmetrical, usually oval. The central pigmented naevus may slowly disappear and there is usually gradual repigmentation of the halo. These appearances must be distinguished from depigmentation around a malignant melanoma. In this example a pigmented compound naevus (see Fig. 19.3) is surrounded by a symmetrical depigmented zone, in this case probably the result of regression (see below).

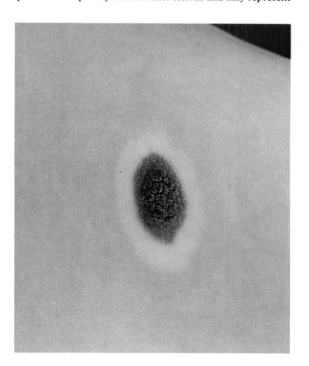

Regression in Naevi

The natural history of many naevi is for reduction in size with age. Histologically, this is usually associated with loss of melanocytes from a lesion, and replacement by fibrosis. In some naevi there is destruction of component melanocytes in association with a chronic inflammatory response in the region of the lesion. Inflammatory cells are lymphocytic with macrophages in the dermis taking up liberated melanin.

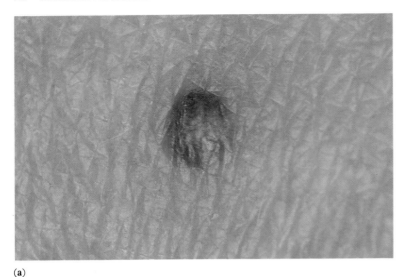

(a)

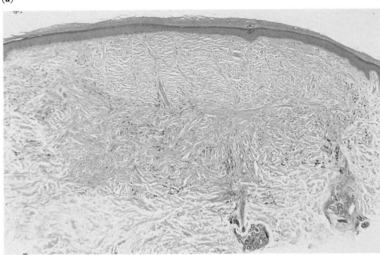

(b)

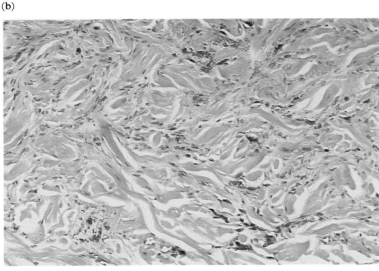

(c)

Fig. 19.6(a), (b) & (c) Blue naevus

Clinically these are domed, smooth-surfaced, blue-grey papules, usually less than 1 cm in diameter. They are commonest on the head and arms, and usually develop in childhood and grow slowly thereafter (a).

The blue naevus is a dermal lesion (b) with a mixture of fine spindle-shaped melanocytes and plump melanin-containing macrophages separated by haphazard collagen bundles (c). Histologically these lesions can be confused with a dermatofibroma containing iron pigment. The melanin pigment in the melanocytes may be difficult to see as it is finely dispersed; it can be better seen with a special stain for melanin. The blue, rather than brown, colour of these lesions clinically results from the optical effect of their location in the dermis.

Large blue naevi, often greater than 1 cm in diameter, are usually found on the buttocks and perineum. Histologically, they are distinct because they are made up of rounded fascicles and bundles of plump spindle-shaped cells. These cells may contain little melanin, which is more easily seen in small aggregates of macrophages scattered throughout the tumour. This variant is described as cellular blue naevus by pathologists. Most of these lesions behave in a benign manner despite the occasional presence of cellular atypia. Very rarely, metastasis can occur with some of these atypical lesions (malignant blue naevus), and such behaviour can be almost impossible to predict on histological grounds as there is little histological difference between this and a benign cellular blue naevus with cellular atypia; the presence of increased mitotic activity and abnormal mitoses sometimes helps. There is similarity between cellular blue naevi and pigment-containing nerve sheath tumours. Naevus of Ota is a blue naevus in the area of the trigeminal nerve. Naevus of Ito is a blue naevus in the acromio-clavicular region.

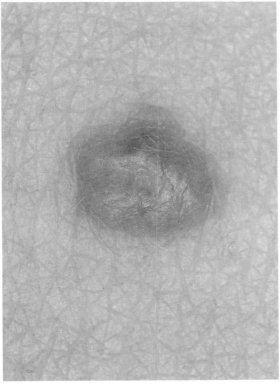

(a)

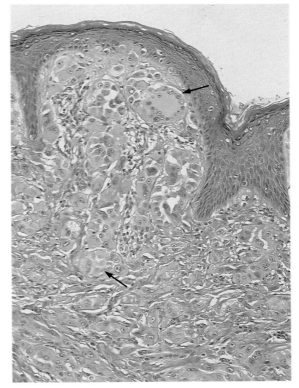

(b)

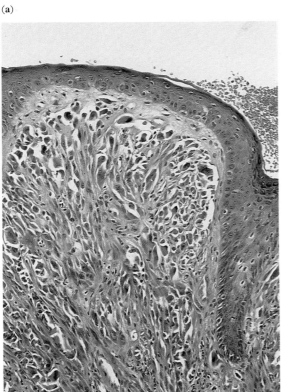

(c)

Fig. 19.7(a), (b) & (c) Juvenile melanoma (Spitz naevus)

Clinically, juvenile melanomas present as oval, well-defined, domed and smooth papules with a red-brown colour (a). It is unusual to find pigment variegation. They are commonest in children but may occur at any age. Histological identification of this lesion is often difficult because of similarities with the features of malignant melanoma. Fortunately it is clinically distinct but in children may be clinically confused with juvenile xanthogranuloma (see Fig. 23.4) or mast cell tumour (see Fig. 13.2a), although the latter urticates on rubbing. The lesion is best regarded as a proliferating variant of compound naevus. The melanocytes may be junctional, intra-epidermal or intradermal. These cells are arranged in irregular nests and there are usually two cell types: fascicles of epithelioid cells which have plump voluminous cytoplasm with multinucleate forms (arrows in (b)), and spindle shaped cells (c). The cells deeper in the lesion tend to be smaller and more compact and are surrounded by a lymphocytic infiltrate. A noteworthy feature is the presence of large dilated capillary vessels in the upper part of the lesion with oedema of stroma and separation of melanocyte nests by loose connective tissue. Mitotic figures are common in this type of lesion but do not indicate malignancy.

The histological recognition of this entity depends on awareness of the possibility and positive searching for the combination of oedema, capillary vessels and lymphocytic infiltration in the presence of an appropriate cellularity to the melanocytic nests.

Malignant Melanoma

There is epidemiological evidence that the incidence of malignant melanoma is increasing in many parts of the world.

The clinical hallmarks of malignant melanoma are irregularity of edge (e.g. notching), colour and surface. It is said that skin lines are lost in melanoma but this is an unreliable sign. Also lesions can be amelanotic and lack pigment. Fortunately total loss of pigment is rare and so the diagnosis is usually apparent.

Clinically and pathologically, it is common practice to divide malignant melanoma into one of four types: lentigo maligna melanoma; superficial spreading malignant melanoma; nodular malignant melanoma; acral lentiginous malignant melanoma.

Histologically and clinically, several features serve to subdivide and distinguish these types from each other; these are site, lateral growth, and vertical growth.

Site:

Lentigo maligna melanoma usually occurs on the face, and acral lentiginous malignant melanomas occur on the palms, soles and mucosae. Nodular malignant melanoma and superficial spreading malignant melanoma may occur in any site.

Lateral and vertical growth phases:

Histopathologically, an important prognostic feature appears to be whether the melanocytic lesion has a growth phase which is lateral or vertical. In the same way that a tree may either have a deep tap root (vertical growth phase) or a spreading superficial root system (lateral growth phase), so a malignant melanoma may show either of these patterns, or both. (text continues on opposite page)

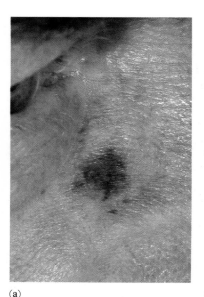

(a)

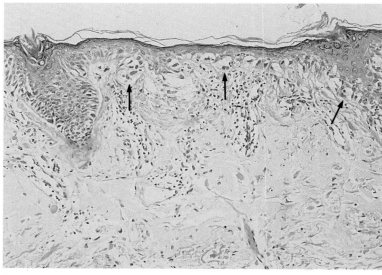

(b)

Fig. 19.8(a) & (b) Lentigo maligna (Hutchinson's freckle)

Clinically, this presents as variegated, macular, brown-black pigmentation, usually on the face in the elderly (a). There is a sharp outline with a notched irregular border. Lesions may be several centimetres in diameter; sometimes there are papules within the macule (see below).

Histologically, the epidermis is thinned and may be atrophic (b). There is replacement of the basal layer of the epidermis by pleomorphic melanocytes (arrows), varying from small cells to large cells with rounded hyperchromatic nuclei and large red-staining nucleoli. Mitoses may be seen in these cells. While most of the basal layer is replaced in a virtually continuous fashion, small discontinuities may be seen, corresponding with the paler areas seen clinically. There is no evidence of a breach in the basal lamina and hence the atypical melanocytes are confined to the

epidermis where the lesion is localized as an in situ atypical melanocytic proliferation. Cells may extend down along the root sheath of hair follicles and sweat glands, but this should not be interpreted as invasion, although they may be apparent clinically as papules within the otherwise flat lesion. Pigment is seen within macrophages in the upper dermis and a variable upper dermal lymphocytic infiltrate is a frequent accompaniment to the lesion.

Late lesions develop junctional clusters of atypical melanocytes and it is at this stage that invasive growth is most likely to be present. The presence of clusters of atypical cells in the epidermis of a lentigo maligna should prompt a careful search for invasive tumour. This often starts in areas around hair follicles.

As with any melanocytic lesion, changes of regression may complicate the histological picture.

In the *lateral growth phase* there is growth of the lesion along or parallel with the epidermis. This is the pattern of growth shown by lentigo maligna, superficial spreading malignant melanoma, and acral lentiginous melanoma but not nodular malignant melanoma. Whilst the growth phase remains lateral, the prognosis appears to be good, providing the lesions are completely excised. However, in all of the above examples, a vertical growth phase may supervene and the prognosis worsen.

In the *vertical growth phase* there is growth of the lesion down into the dermis, and the prognosis is worse than in lesions with lateral growth phase only. If a vertical growth pattern is present without any detectable lateral growth, then this is nodular malignant melanoma (see Fig. 19.11).

A vertical growth phase may supervene in any of the lesions in which the growth phase had formerly been exclusively lateral. In lentigo maligna, this is manifest by the development of a nodule in the previously flat lesion, the nodule representing the area undergoing a vertical growth phase; this is called *lentigo maligna melanoma*. (see Fig. 19.9). The complete assessment of prognosis in malignant melanoma depends largely on histological evaluation of the excised lesion, and will be considered after discussing these four types of lesion.

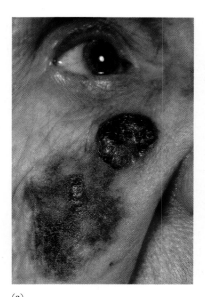

(a)

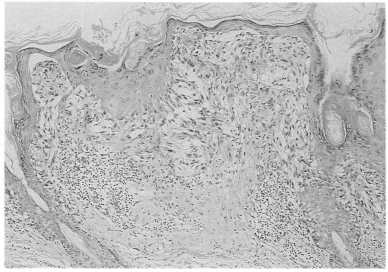

(b)

Fig. 19.9(a) & (b) Lentigo maligna melanoma and acral lentigenous melanoma

After many years, an invasive vertical growth phase may develop in a lentigo maligna (lentigo maligna melanoma). This usually appears as a nodule, often darkly and variably pigmented, sometimes ulcerating (a).

Histologically, an area of invasive melanoma extending into the dermis is seen arising within a lateral growth pattern lentigo maligna. The invasive component often begins around hair follicles (b) as an extension of the intra-epidermal clusters seen in the late lesion (see Fig. 19.8(b)). The atypical invasive melanocytes are frequently spindle cell in shape and are associated with dermal collagen, giving rise to cells infiltrating between dense collagen bundles (desmoplastic melanoma).

In assessing the lesions, the depth of invasion should be recorded from histological section (see Fig. 19.14, p.151), as should the completeness of excision laterally and deeply.

Acral lentigenous malignant melanoma is commonest in negroes, Asians and orientals; it is rarely seen in the UK. Clinically and histologically, it shows very similar features to those described above for lentigo maligna malignant melanoma.

Superficial spreading malignant melanoma

The term superficial spreading malignant melanoma often causes confusion, as it is sometimes used synonymously with in-situ malignant melanoma; however, the terms are not interchangeable. Superficial spreading malignant melanoma can be either in situ (confined to the epidermis) or invasive (where it extends into the dermis).

Histologically, the lesion shows large, lightly pigmented atypical melanocytes forming clusters and disposed singly at all levels in the epidermis. If this change is confined to the epidermis after a careful search of several histological slides of the lesion, then it may be termed *in-situ superficial spreading malignant melanoma* (formerly pagetoid malignant melanoma in-situ). A lymphocytic response in the upper dermis is a common accompaniment to the lesion, along with pigment-containing dermal macrophages.

Invasive superficial spreading malignant melanoma is the more usual form of this tumour. The invasive component is formed of nests of cells growing into the dermis. The nests in the upper dermis are frequently of the same size as the epidermal nests (10–15 cells across) and the cells are of similar type. This has been taken to suggest an early form of invasion of a tumour in a radial (predominantly lateral) growth phase. The emergence of large invasive nests of cells which are larger and more pleomorphic than the epidermal component heralds the vertical growth phase of the tumour, when metastatic spread is more likely. These large solid nests of atypical invasive cells result in thicker lesions, that is, those associated with a poorer prognosis. Lymphocytic infiltration, pigment-containing macrophages in the dermis, and ulceration are common accompanying features.

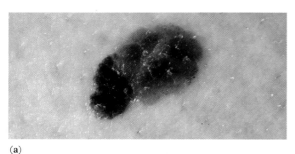

(a)

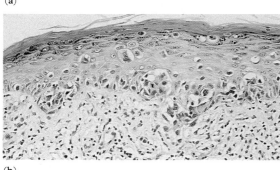

(b)

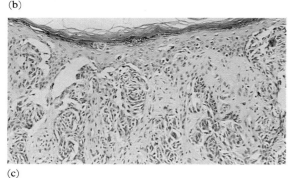

(c)

Fig. 19.10(a), (b) & (c) Superficial spreading malignant melanoma

Clinically, the lesion is smaller than lentigo maligna but has a similar irregular notched outline and pigment variegation from brown to black(a). Bluish-grey discolouration implies that there is melanin in the dermis and hence suggests vertical invasion. The edge is often palpable and the lesion usually contains raised areas, either nodules or papules. Lesions occur anywhere on the trunk or limbs.

In micrograph (b), an example of superficial spreading malignant melanoma in situ, note the discontinuous replacement of the basal layer of the epidermis by nests of melanocytes and also single cells. There are also cells high up in the epidermis as single cells with clear spaces around them and small groups of two or three cells. At higher magnification, these cells have pleomorphic nuclei with hyperchromatism and prominent nucleoli. Mitotic figures are visible. Such features identify the melanocytes as atypical. A lymphocytic dermal infiltrate is often present at the base of the lesion.

The separation of this entity from other atypical melanocytic proliferations can be difficult. Identification of discontinuous basal cell replacement and upward invasion of the epidermis are the criteria for identifying a lesion as malignant melanoma in situ rather than a lesser degree of atypical proliferation such as a dysplastic naevus (see Fig. 19.13).

In micrograph (c), an example of invasive superficial spreading malignant melanoma, there is an area of early invasive melanoma arising by dermal invasion occurring in a previously in situ lesion.

Comparison of the nests of melanocytes in the invasive vertical growth component and the epidermal junctional (lateral) component reveals in most cases that the invasive cells are larger, with clear cytoplasm, and in nests which are larger and more irregular than the junctional nests.

Nodular malignant melanoma

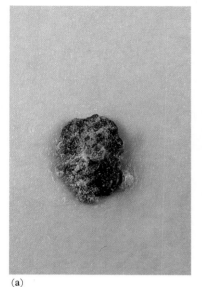

(a)

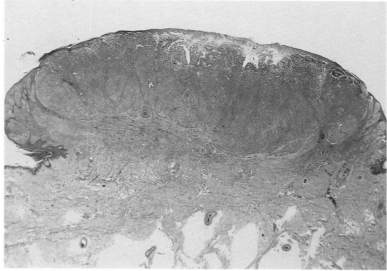

(b)

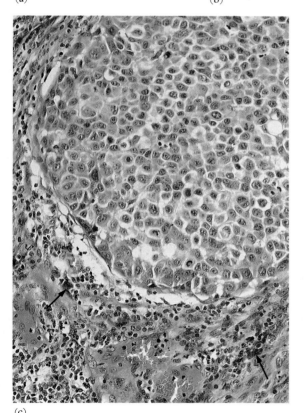

(c)

Fig. 19.11(a), (b) & (c) Nodular malignant melanoma
Unlike the two previous forms, lesions are always raised
throughout, either as a nodule or a plaque. Often there is
pigment variegation suggestive of malignancy, with colour
ranging from red to black. Depigmentation also occurs as
with other forms, and lesions can be uniformly black like a
berry (a). Lesions often grow rapidly and frequently
ulcerate.

A nodular malignant melanoma has no lateral growth
phase. The cellular nests which form the invasive tumour
tend to be larger than the superficial nests of a superficial
spreading malignant melanoma, frequently forming a
polypoid nodule invading the dermis (b). Cells show
pleomorphism and may be epithelioid or spindle cell in
type; micrograph (c) shows a large invasive dermal nodule
of epithelioid malignant melanocytes with surrounding
reactive lymphocytic infiltration.

Melanin is present in dermal macrophages both within
and around the lesion (arrows), the melanocytes only
showing melanin in occasional cells. Both spindle cell and
epithelioid cell patterns occur in invasive nodular
melanoma; the spindle cell component may simulate other
spindle cell tumours.

The concept of separating the nodular malignant
melanoma from other types may be artificial in that the
nodular type may have arisen in another lesion but rapid
growth may have destroyed a pre-existing, in situ
component. It merely implies that no in situ component is
identifiable at the time of diagnosis.

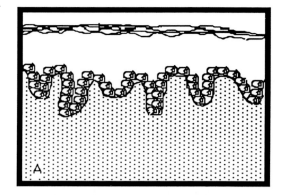

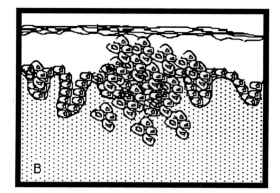

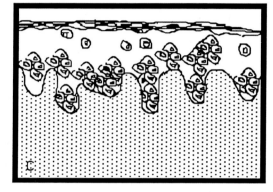

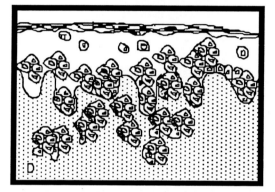

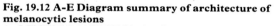

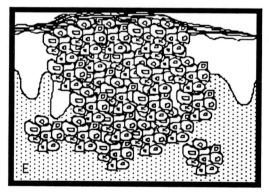

Fig. 19.12 A-E Diagram summary of architecture of melanocytic lesions

A. LENTIGO MALIGNA showing only lateral growth phase.
B. LENTIGO MALIGNA MELANOMA showing additional vertical growth phase.
C. SUPERFICIAL SPREADING MALIGNANT MELANOMA IN SITU showing extension of melanocytes singly and in clumps into upper epidermal layers.
D. INVASIVE SUPERFICIAL SPREADING MALIGNANT MELANOMA with additional vertical growth phase.
E. NODULAR MALIGNANT MELANOMA with no lateral growth phase but vertical growth phase both upwards through epidermis and downwards invading dermis.

Borderline malignant melanocytic lesions

The diagnosis of invasive malignant melanoma is often difficult, especially in assessing junctional activity in a compound naevus which has clinically been enlarging or becoming more pigmented. Upward extension of melanocytes into the epidermis, forming small clumps of cells cut off from the epidermal nests is a feature suggesting malignant melanoma. With regard to identifying an invasive component, a change of character of the melanocytes in the invasive nests is also helpful. A lymphocytic inflammatory flare around a melanotic lesion should always give rise to consideration of whether the lesion is malignant melanoma although this sign is unreliable since regressing melanocytic lesions of all types may show lymphocytic infiltrate.

A lesion which often causes diagnostic difficulty is the so-called dysplastic naevus.

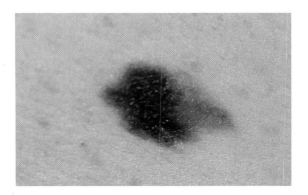

(a)

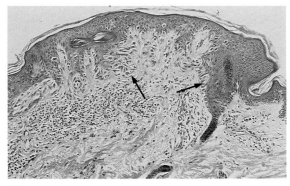

(b)

Fig. 19.13(a) & (b) Dysplastic naevus
These are naevi which clinically have one or several features suggesting malignancy. They are often large (greater than 1 cm diameter) with some irregularity of edge, colour and surface (a). They occur at any site; often one individual has several. Usually they increase in number with age but some may be congenital. Frequently, they run in families and there may be a history of relatives with malignant melanoma. The risk of malignant melanoma is increased in these individuals; however, tumours arise from normal-looking skin as well as from the naevi.

Dysplastic naevi may have junctional and dermal components. The problem arises when one component is inappropriate in cytology or architectural arrangement. *Atypia of a junctional component* is identified as irregular proliferation of junctional melanocytes discontinuously and irregularly spaced along the dermo-epidermal junction. Occasional cells in the melanocytic proliferation will show large nuclei with a big nucleolus and coarse chromatin indicative of an atypical nuclear cytology. Another helpful feature for identifying atypical junctional proliferation is lack of roundness of the nests of cells, which tend to be flat and follow the general contour of the epidermal rete ridges, as in micrograph (arrows in (b)).

Clumps of isolated melanocytes spreading up through the epidermis is not a feature of this condition but identifies in situ superficial spreading malignant melanoma; a careful search for this feature is mandatory in all atypical melanocytic lesions.

Atypia of the dermal component may also occur. This is manifest by occasional cells in dermal nests having atypical large or hyperchromatic nuclei. Architecturally, the nests of dermal melanocytes are irregularly spaced in the dermis and are of unequal size, orientation, and shape, tending to lack the spherical nesting structure of a simple compound naevus. Diagnostic difficulty may be found in deciding whether a lesion is invasive malignant melanoma. Nests of cells forming the invasive component of malignant melanoma frequently differ from the cytology of junctional melanocytes or the epidermal component, and most cells are atypical as opposed to only a proportion of cells in a dysplastic naevus. Architecturally, the dermal invasive nests of malignant melanoma tend to be larger and much more irregular than the epidermal nests. Despite these helpful features, the classification of a lesion as malignant melanoma or atypical (dysplastic) naevus may be very difficult.

Prognostic features in malignant melanoma

Several clinical and pathological features of primary cutaneous malignant melanoma may be used to assess the risk of local recurrence or metastasis following excision. Of these, by far the best single predictor is thickness.

The *Breslow thickness assessment* (see Fig. 19.14(a)) is made on paraffin sections by direct measurement of tumour thickness perpendicular to the epidermis at the maximum depth of tumour. This is done using an eyepiece graticule or a vernier scale on a microscope stage. Measurement is from the granular layer of the epidermis to the deepest, easily identifiable tumour cell in the dermis beneath. The thicker the tumour, the worse the five-year survival. A cut-off of thickness may be used to divide lesions into good, intermediate and poor prognosis. Lesions less than 1.5 mm thick have a greater than 90% five-year survival; those with a thickness greater than 1.5 mm, but less than 3.0 mm have a greater than 60% five-year survival, whilst lesions thicker than 3.0 mm have 40% five-year survival. The other system, often used in conjunction with Breslow thickness, is Clarke's level.

For the *Clarke level*, the depth within the dermis to which the melanoma extends determines the stage: this is shown diagrammatically in Figure 19.14(b).

While the Clarke level and Breslow thickness are useful guides to likely outcome, they are not absolute and are subject to sampling error (shrinkage artefact, taking the right block, orientating the skin, measuring accurately) and intra- and interobserver errors as to which is the greatest depth, what is perpendicular to the skin surface, and where is the start of the reticular dermis? Clearly, completeness of excision is crucial and vascular or lymphatic invasion are important. It is important in this respect to sample edges of resection margins and several areas of a lesion, particularly flat macular lesions which have been excised because of pigment change or growth. After formalin fixation, any slight pigment variegation or small papular zones in a flat melanotic lesion may not be appreciated by the pathologist cutting up the specimen. A small drawing of the lesion indicating the suspect areas will direct block sampling or the need to sample at several histological levels. In this way atypical foci or early in situ change will not be missed and, more importantly, early invasion at one margin of a small lesion will not go unsampled.

These factors should be considered when planning treatment and giving advice about an excised lesion.

Conventional histological features of malignancy such as extreme pleomorphism, high mitotic rate, and nuclear hyperchromatism are generally associated with an aggressive lesion; however, prognosis is best related to the tumour size (assessed by thickness).

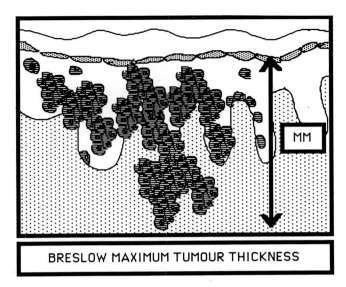

BRESLOW MAXIMUM TUMOUR THICKNESS

Fig. 19.14(a) Breslow tumour thickness.

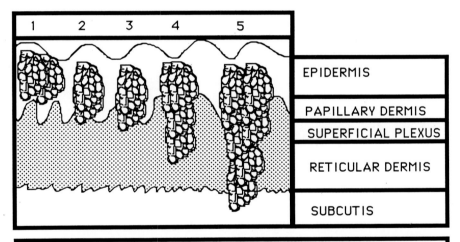

1	2	3	4	5

EPIDERMIS

PAPILLARY DERMIS

SUPERFICIAL PLEXUS

RETICULAR DERMIS

SUBCUTIS

Clarke level 1	Confined to epidermis
Clarke level 2	Invasion into papillary dermis
Clarke level 3	Involvement of superficial vascular plexus
Clarke level 4	Invasion of the reticular dermis
Clarke level 5	Invasion of the Subcutaneous tissues

Fig. 19.14 (b) Clarke levels for malignant melanoma.

20. Epithelial skin appendage hamartomas and tumours

Introduction

The epithelial skin appendages comprise the pilosebaceous apparatus, eccrine sweat gland and duct, and apocrine sweat gland and duct. Abnormal overgrowths of these are common, and can be subdivided into hamartomatous malformations and true neoplasms, athough in some instances the distinction is not always clear. The most frequent hamartomous malformations of skin appendages are accessory nipple and naevus sebaceous; the epidermal naevus is a hamartomatous malformation of surface epidermis alone but is considered here for convenience.

Most skin appendage tumours behave in a benign fashion and rarely metastasize, although they tend to recur if incompletely excised. Some examples are multifocal (e.g. trichoepithelioma, cylindroma). Skin appendage tumours which are malignant from the outset are rare.

Skin appendage hamartomas

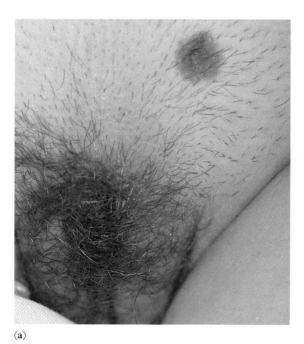

(a)

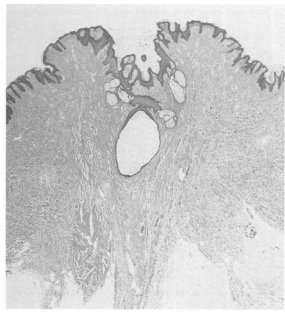

(b)

Fig. 20.1(a) & (b). Accessory nipple

The breast is a specialized sweat gland with a large and complex secretory lobular gland component and a prominent branching duct system opening to the exterior at the nipple; both lobular and duct system are hormone-dependent, developing and secreting under hormonal stimulus. The male breast remains rudimentary, with non-development of the lobular system and variable persistence of a usually non-branching duct system.

Accessory nipples can occur anywhere along the embryological 'milk-line', an oblique line extending from the anterior margin of the axilla and running obliquely down across the chest and abdomen to the groin on the same side, and terminating on the medial aspect of the thigh. The

majority occur on the chest and abdomen, and are most frequent near the true nipple; they can occasionally be multiple and bilateral. Clinically, they appear as 0.5–1 cm brown papules with various degrees of semblance to normal nipples; the brown skin is usually wrinkled, with a protuberant centre in which open pores can be seen. Histologically, they appear as rudimentary nipples, with a number of immature lactiferous ducts and, rarely, deeper secretory lobules. Bundles of smooth muscle are prominent around the ducts in the upper dermis. The overlying epidermis is irregularly acanthotic and hyperkeratotic. Accessory nipples may become more prominent in pregnancy, with duct dilatation and duct epithelial hyperplasia.

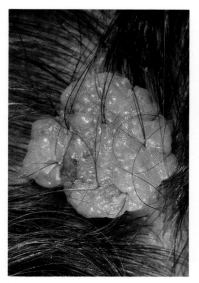

(a)

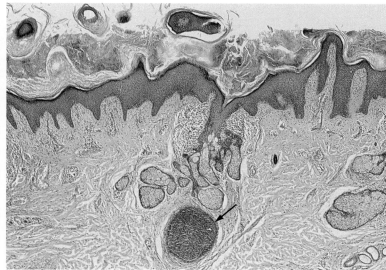

(b)

Fig. 20.2 (a), (b) & (c). Naevus sebaceous (organoid naevus)
These are present at birth, and are most common in the scalp, but occasionally occur on the neck and face. Despite their name, sebaceous glands are not always the most prominent feature, and the histological appearances vary with the age of the patient. Clinically, they appear as usually oval or linear raised plaques with a somewhat bosselated yellowish surface with a waxy feel; when arising in the scalp they are relatively hairless (a). In children they are usually flatter and smoother because sebaceous hypertrophy is androgen-dependent. Appendageal tumours may develop occasionally in a naevus sebaceous; syringocystadenoma, developing from the apocrine component, is the most frequent. Basal and squamous cell carcinomas, and appendageal carcinomas, can also develop. This change usually occurs in adult life, and is frequent enough to justify prophylactic excision.

The histological appearance is very variable but two constant features are structural abnormalities of the pilosebaceous apparatus, and of overlying surface epidermis. Other frequent findings are dilated sweat glands and ducts. In infancy and childhood (as in (b)), a prominent feature is the presence of numerous immature hair germ clusters composed of basal cells (arrow), and resembling small islands of basal cell carcinoma but with evidence of primitive follicle or sebaceous differentiation. Sebaceous differentiation is particularly prominent after puberty, but the

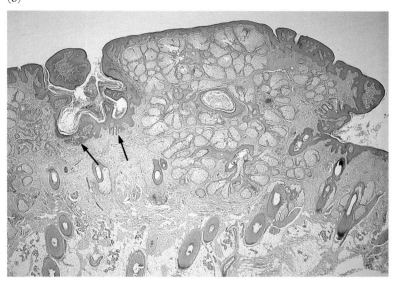

(c)

glands are disordered and show abnormal relationship with such hair follicles as are present, and may be very superficial, sometimes opening directly onto the skin surface. Hair follicle formation is similarly disordered, and normal follicles containing hair shafts are rare, hence the 'baldness' of the lesion; most attempts at hair follicle formation result in distended, keratin-filled tubes or cysts. Although comparatively scarce in infants (when primitive hair germ islands are frequent), this maturation into architecturally abnormal pilosebaceous components becomes the major feature in adult life and dominates the histological picture

as in (c), although a careful search usually reveals some immature hair germ islands, particularly at the periphery of the lesion; see arrows in (c). Pathologists should examine a number of blocks of large lesions to get a true picture of the proportions of the various components present, taking particular care to examine the edges of the lesion; if immature hair germ islands are frequent, and particularly if they are interconnected with each other and with the overlying epidermis, then deeper levels should be examined to exclude the development of basal cell carcinoma.

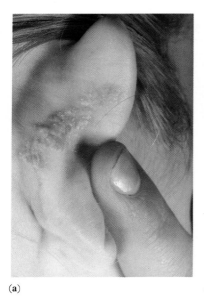

(a)

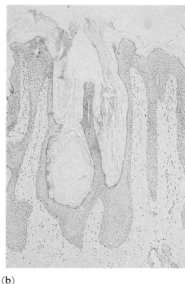

(b)

Fig. 20.3(a) & (b). Epidermal naevus

Verrucous epidermal naevi present as initially flat, then increasingly warty lines or whorled streaks of hyperkeratosis (a). They usually become apparent soon after birth. Inflammatory epidermal naevi have a similar linear disposition, but consist of red scaly papules with a sharp outline, usually on the leg and thigh. In the more common warty (verrucous) pattern, the histological changes are acanthosis, papillomatosis and focal hypergranulosis, with overlying hyperkeratosis (b), somewhat resembling a viral wart in architecture but without the cytological changes of virus-infected cells (compare with Fig. 10.2(c)). In the flatter, plaque-like lesions, the histological changes resemble those of a seborrhoeic keratosis. Inflammatory epidermal naevi show spongiosis and inflammatory cell infiltrate of epidermis and dermis in addition to the epidermal changes described above.

SKIN APPENDAGE TUMOURS

True skin appendage tumours can usually be classified according to their presumed tissue of origin.

Tumours derived from pilosebaceous unit

Fig. 20.4. Trichofolliculoma

This lesion appears as a small pearly nodule, approximately the same colour as surrounding skin, with a central pit from which a cluster of fine white hairs may protrude. They are almost always solitary and are confined to the head and neck, most commonly the face. A lesion which is clinically similar, but largely confined to the skin of the upper lip, is the pilar sheath acanthoma. Both trichofolliculoma and pilar sheath acanthoma are found in adults.

Histologically, a large dilated hair follicle lined by squamous epithelium extends into the dermis. Occasionally, the surface connection is not seen and a keratinized squamous-lined cyst results. Radiating from this 'primary follicle' are numerous buds of basaloid cells which form small 'secondary follicles', some of which may contain a fine hair shaft. Occasional secondary follicle buds contain a small horn cyst reminiscent of trichoepithelioma (see Fig. 20.5).

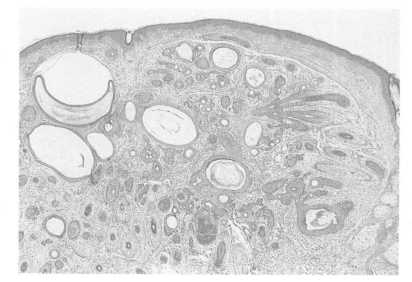

Fig. 20.5. Trichoepithelioma

Multiple lesions are inherited as an autosomal dominant disorder, and occur on the central face at puberty. They begin as 1–2 mm papules and increase in size with age. There may be prominent surface telangiectasia, and ulceration suggests the development of basal cell carcinoma.

Isolated lesions are much more common and are not inherited. They are most common on the face of teenagers and young adults, and present as a skin-coloured nodule up to 1 cm in diameter. There may be a central shallow depression but no true pit (cf. trichofolliculoma).

Histologically, small nests and cords of basaloid cells reminiscent of basal cell carcinoma are seen, with some of the nests having horn cysts with abrupt keratinization (arrow). In many lesions, rudimentary hair papillae are seen formed from the basaloid nests. This tumour merges in appearance with basal cell carcinoma with keratotic horn cysts. Large proportions of basaloid cells, small numbers of horn cysts and lack of primitive hair papillae would suggest keratotic basal cell carcinoma rather

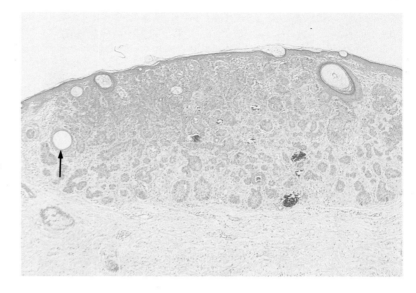

than trichoepithelioma. Desmoplastic trichoepithelioma is characterized by compression of the basaloid nests and horn cysts by dermal fibrous proliferation. The presence of keratin horn cysts allows distinction of this tumour from similar syringoma (cysts lined by a double layer epithelium) and morphoeic basal cell carcinoma where horn cysts are rarely seen.

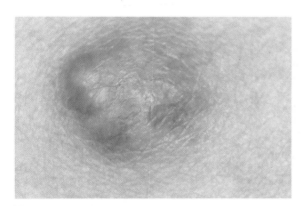

(a)

(b)

Fig. 20.6(a) & (b). Pilomatrixoma (calcifying epithelioma of Malherbe)

This is a tumour composed of primitive basaloid cells showing evidence of differentiation towards hair matrix production.

They occur mainly in children and are most common on the face, neck, shoulders and arms. They are almost always solitary and knobbly dermal or subcutaneous tumours with a bluish tinge (a). Most are 1–2 cm in diameter.

Histology of these lesions varies according to the degree of maturation of the tumour and whether sufficient time has elapsed for calcification and other degenerative phenomena to occur. The proliferating cells are seen as irregular islands of dark-staining basaloid cells which instead of maturing to keratinization, become eosinophilic and have a central lucent zone representing the lost nucleus (b). These pale eosinophilic areas are termed 'shadow cells' (arrow). Calcification, and a brisk foreign body giant cell reaction to the hair-matrix material, frequently dominate the histology of an old or traumatized lesion, and a careful search for the shadow cell component is often needed to diagnose the lesion, as basaloid cells are not present in older lesions.

Other hair-follicle related tumours

Inverted follicular keratosis is the name given to a lesion in which there is an adenomatous proliferation of cells related to follicular sheath epithelium. It is seen on the face in middle-aged patients as a yellowish papule with a central plug of keratin. Histologically, there is hyper- and parakeratosis over a lesion composed of basaloid cells with central eddies of maturation to cells resembling the prickle cell layer of epidermis. The lesion extends from epidermis as finger-like downgrowths into the dermis. There is some debate as to whether this lesion is a genuine adenoma or whether it represents an irritated seborrhoeic keratosis, which is also a lesion composed of basaloid cells and squamous eddies; see Figure 17.3(c).

Trichilemmoma is most common in the elderly and is a solitary pinkish or brown nodule on the face, usually about 0.5 cm in diameter which resembles a basal cell carcinoma. Histologically, the lesion is seen as lobulated flowing sheets of cells extending from the lower part of the epidermis into the dermis. At the periphery of the cellular sheets there is a zone of nuclear palisading reminiscent of basal cell carcinoma which separates this entity from the similar low magnification architecture seen in eccrine poroma and clonal seborrhoeic keratosis. A thick PAS-positive membrane is seen around the islands of cells comprising this tumour.

The *dilated pore of Winer* is a solitary lesion, usually on the face of adult males, and resembles a large comedo, being rounded and having a central pit which is plugged with a horny mass of dark keratin. Histologically, there is apparent invagination of the epidermis to line a pit filled with keratin. The lesion is thought to represent an adenomatous proliferation of the infundibular portion of hair follicle. The epithelium lining the pit is irregular and may have small buds growing into the dermis. Marsupialization of an epidermal cyst may result in a similar lesion. If basaloid buds with follicular differentiation are present around the central pit then trichofolliculoma should be considered. Proliferation of lobulated cell masses from around a central pit or cyst should also bring to mind the possibility of a pilar sheath acanthoma, a lesion seen usually on the lip.

Hair follicle cysts

Cysts are common lesions in the skin, most commonly derived from the hair follicle structures.

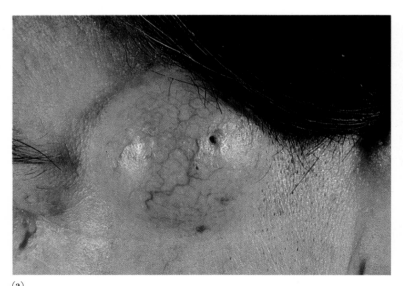

(a)

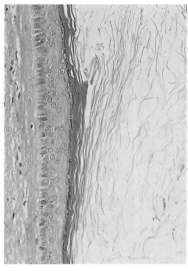

(b)

Fig. 20.7(a) & (b) Epidermal cyst

These present as mobile, rounded, subcutaneous nodules over which the skin is stretched thin. There may be a central punctum (a) through which some of the cyst's 'cheesy' contents may extrude. They may occur anywhere, but are common on the face; in other sites, they may follow trauma and implantation of epidermis (inclusion epidermal cyst).

They are histologically characterized by a wall lined by squamous epithelium with keratinization via a granular layer. The central portion of the cyst contains pink-staining keratin. A frequently seen feature is a foreign body reaction with histiocytic giant cells either within the cyst or more usually around the cyst. This foreign body inflammatory response is usually due to traumatic cyst rupture and is often clinically interpreted as 'infected' epidermal cyst. The common use of the term sebaceous cyst is incorrect as this type of cyst does not have anything to do with sebaceous glands.

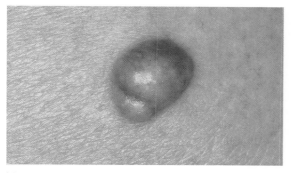

(a)

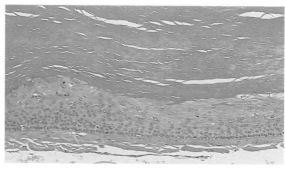

(b)

Fig. 20.8(a) & (b). Pilar (trichilemmal) cysts

These are clinically similar to epidermal cysts (a) but are usually confined to the scalp; they are frequently multiple, and in some cases are familial.

Histologically, they are epidermal cysts with pilar (hair follicle) type of keratinization without a granular layer. They have a wall of squamous epithelium and abrupt

keratinization with loss of nuclei, eosinophilia and rounding of cells towards the surface of the epithelium. The central keratin may show focal calcification which is seen as blue-stained irregular masses on H & E sections. A foreign body inflammatory reaction may be an associated feature as with epidermal cysts.

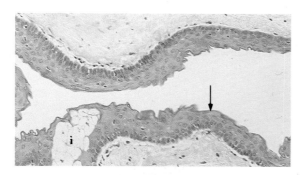

Fig. 20.9. Steatocystoma multiplex

In this condition there are cysts derived from the entire pilosebaceous unit. It is an autosomal dominant inherited disorder which presents at around puberty with the appearance of large numbers of smooth rubbery round nodules in the skin of the trunk and limbs.

Histologically the cysts are thin-walled. The main diagnostic feature is a thin brightly eosinophilic, almost glassy, band of keratin lining the cyst, with underlying flattened squamous cells (arrow). Careful examination often shows flattened foamy cells of a sebaceous gland (i) in part of the cyst wall. Occasional small multiple vellus-like hair shafts may be present in the cyst contents.

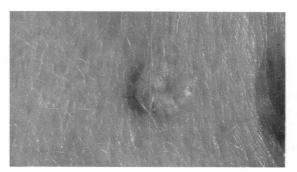

(a)

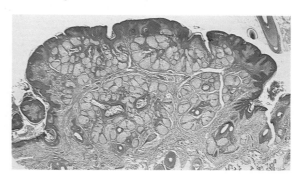

(b)

Fig. 20.10(a) & (b). Sebaceous hyperplasia, adenoma, and carcinoma

Sebaceous adenoma is a rare solitary tumour which must be differentiated clinically and histologically from sebaceous hyperplasia which is exceedingly common. Sebaceous carcinoma is very rare.

In *sebaceous hyperplasia*, there are usually a number of 2–5 mm yellow telangiectatic umbilicated papules, most commonly on the forehead and cheeks of middle-aged and elderly people; occasionally solitary lesions occur and can be confused with basal cell carcinoma (a).

In sebaceous hyperplasia, large lipid-predominant sebaceous lobules surround a central duct, with few peripheral germinative cells (b).

Sebaceous adenoma is usually larger, and is a firm, warty-surfaced, yellowish papule. Histologically, there is a lobular arrangement of sebaceous glands in the dermis. The cells in the lobules are composed of peripheral germinative cells having no lipid vacuolation, and more central lipid-rich cells. The term sebaceous epithelioma has been used to describe lesions with less than 50% of cells in the tumour showing lipid vacuolation and many more solid nests of germinative cells, implying a tumour with less differentiation than the adenoma.

Sebaceous carcinoma is briefly discussed on page 163.

TUMOURS DERIVED FROM ECCRINE SWEAT GLANDS

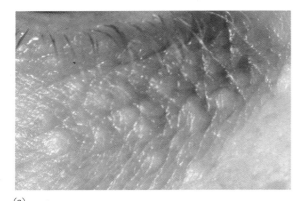

(a)

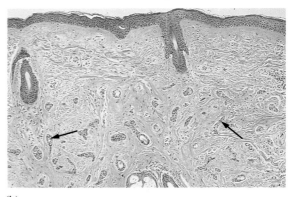

(b)

Fig. 20.11(a) & (b). Syringoma

Syringomas usually appear as grouped, 2–3 mm diameter, flesh-coloured or ivory papules on the lower eyelids (a) and cheeks, most commonly in women. Less commonly they are found as multiple lesions (eruptive syringoma) on the chest and abdomen.

They consist of small proliferated ducts in the dermis, made up of a two-layered epithelium. The picture is distorted by flattening of some of the ducts between the dermal connective tissues to form slit-like spaces and curvilinear profiles resembling tadpoles and commas (arrows in (b)). Some of the cystic ducts contain eosinophilic secretory material which stains with PAS stain.

In desmoplastic trichoepithelioma, similar cords and cystic structures are seen at low power; however, double cell layered ducts are not present and the cysts of trichoepithelioma are keratinous horn cysts (see Fig. 20.5).

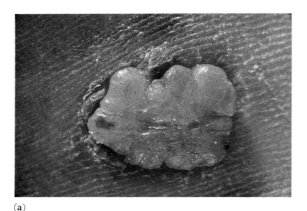

(a)

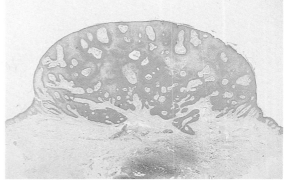

(b)

Fig. 20.12(a), (b) & (c). Eccrine poroma

This is a benign tumour of the epidermal portion of the sweat duct. It presents as a solitary tumour, usually on the sole or palm, as in this example. It is a firm, smooth, pedunculated, 0.5–1 cm bright red nodule which occasionally ulcerates as a result of trauma (a).

At low magnification (b) the lower part of the epidermis is replaced by a lobulated sheet of small cells which extends into the dermis. Separate islands of cells may occur in the dermis, budding off the main mass. The tumour is thus growing from the epidermis. At higher magnification (c), tumour cells can be easily distinguished as uniform oval cells from surrounding epidermis. Occasional slit-like lumina can be seen on careful examination, the lining of which stains with the PAS stain following diastase.

Dermal duct tumour has a similar histology to the eccrine poroma but is intradermal. Confusion may arise between this lesion and basal cell carcinoma, but peripheral palisading is usual in the latter.

Rare examples of malignant eccrine poroma, characterized by marked cellular atypia and metastasis, have been described.

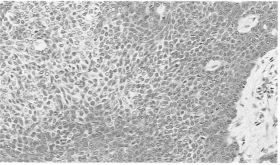

(c)

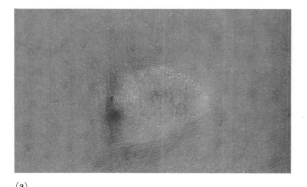

(a)

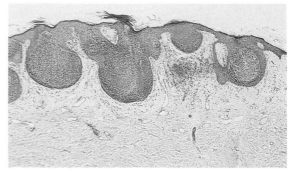

(b)

Fig. 20.13(a) & (b). Hidroacanthoma simplex
This is a benign tumour of intra-epidermal sweat duct origin. The lesion may resemble a seborrhoeic keratosis, except that it is usually present on the lower leg (a). Histologically, the epidermis appears to show irregular thickening at low magnification with large sheets and nests of small cells swelling out from the base of rete ridges and bulging down into the upper dermis (b). The cells at higher power are basaloid cells which contrast with the surrounding prickle cell layer of the epidermis. Dermal invasion is not seen and this tumour is confined to the epidermal layer. This lesion may be considered as an intra-epidermal form of eccrine poroma.

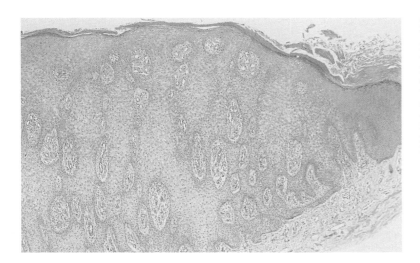

Fig. 20.14. Clear cell acanthoma
This presents as a flat lesion, almost invariably on the legs. Histologically, there is abrupt change in the skin with replacement by an acanthotic epidermis composed of clear cells; these cells contain abundant finely dispersed glycogen, which can be demonstrated by the PAS reaction. A frequent finding is neutrophil polymorphs migrating through the mass of tumour cells.

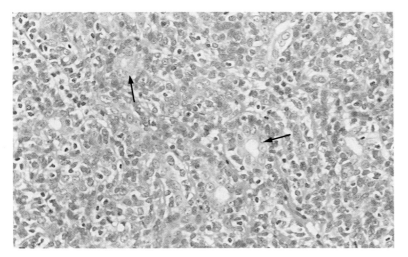

Fig. 20.15. Spiradenoma
This is a tumour of eccrine differentiation with no special site of occurrence. Clinically, it usually arises as a solitary intradermal nodule in early adult life, and can occur anywhere in the body. Most are less than 2 cm in diameter, but occasionally larger examples occur. When multiple, the tumours may be clustered or arranged in a line, rather than scattered. They are frequently tender.

Histologically, they appear as large islands of darkly staining cells in the dermis. On high magnification the islands are made up of large pale cells arranged as a tangle of ducts with small lumina (arrows), with a second population of small dark cells in between. In some examples the lumina are not well-developed.

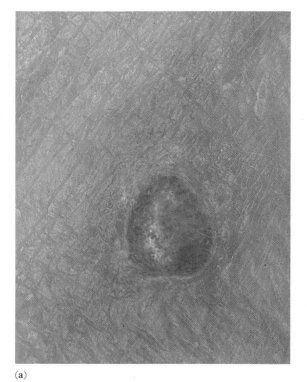

(a)

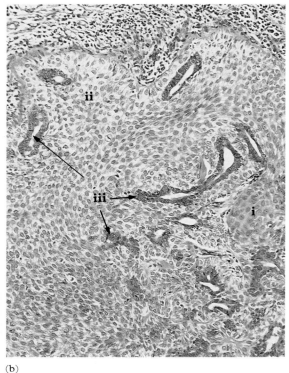

(b)

Fig. 20.16(a) & (b). Clear cell (nodular) hidradenoma
These tumours present as an intradermal nodule usually less than 2 cm in diameter, usually solitary but occasionally multiple. Large lesions may ulcerate.

Histologically, the tumours may be dermal or subcutaneous and are made up of large nodules of cells, often with a surrounding capsule. This type of tumour contains three component cell types. In any individual case, differing proportions of each cell type account for variability in histological pattern from solid to cystic. The cell types demonstrated in micrograph (b) are:

(i) Polyhedral cells with faintly basophilic (purple) cytoplasm and open, round nuclei arranged in sheets and bundles in solid parts of the tumour.

(ii) Rounded large cells with clear cytoplasm which is rich in glycogen, and small, dark-staining nuclei. These are also seen in solid portions of tumour.

(iii) Cuboidal and columnar cells arranged as tubular ducts within the tumour, the lumina of the ducts producing a microcystic appearance.

Solid clear cell tumours exist with few lumina, and were mistakenly called clear cell myoepitheliomas. Most tumours are composed of a mixture of all three cell types as shown here.

These tumours can be considered to be a mixture of eccrine epidermal-ductal, secretory, and dermal-ductal differentiation.

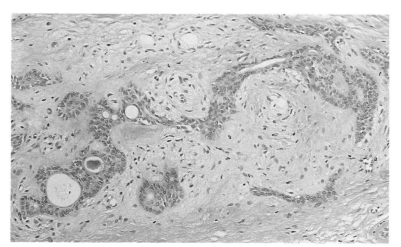

Fig. 20.17. Chondroid syringoma
This tumour resembles the plemorphic salivary adenoma in that it is made up of tubular lumina set in a stroma rich in acid mucopolysaccharides which superficially resembles cartilage.

They are found most commonly on the head and neck as firm, round nodules up to 2 cm in diameter. Since the main tumour mass is dermal, the lesions are covered by intact epidermis.

Histologically, the tumour is composed of small ducts in a branched or tubular pattern, lined by two layers of cells. The stroma is faintly basophilic and contains stellate cells, spindle cells and single epithelial cells. The single cells in the stroma sit in an artifactual lacuna, and hence resemble chondrocytes.

TUMOURS DERIVED FROM APOCRINE SWEAT GLANDS

Fig. 20.18(a), (b) & (c). Apocrine cystadenoma (hidrocystoma)
This usually presents as a solitary cyst on the face, often on the forehead near the eyes (a). The skin is stretched thin over the cyst, and this, combined with the clear fluid contents, gives the lesion a translucent bluish appearance, particularly in large cysts. Smaller cysts do not cause so much thinning of skin and the lesion is more skin-coloured.

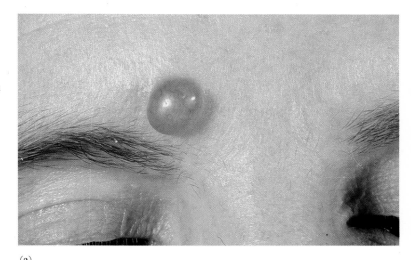

(a)

Histologically (b), these are thin-walled cysts, often collapsed following biopsy (b). The cyst is lined by two layers of cells. The inner columnar layer is an apocrine-type cell layer with pink, tall cells having evidence of the 'decapitation secretion' nipping of apical cytoplasm (c). The outer layer is composed of small dark myoepithelial cells. When the inner layer is cuboidal in type then an eccrine derivation is likely and the lesion is termed eccrine hidrocystoma.

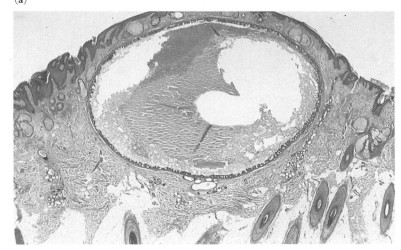

(b)

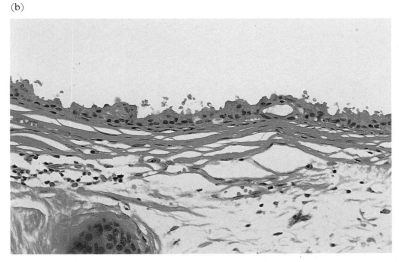

(c)

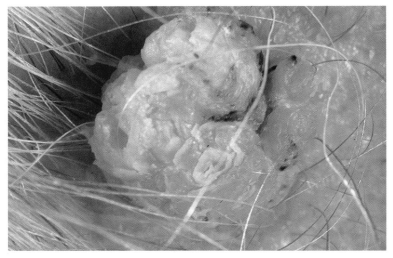

(a)

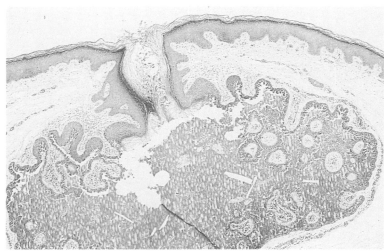

(b)

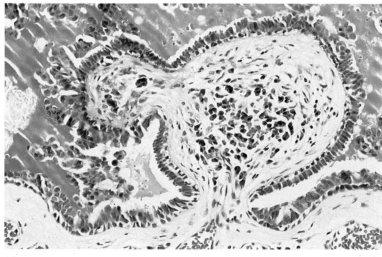

(c)

Fig. 20.19(a), (b) & (c).
Syringocystadenoma papilliferum
This lesion occurs most commonly as benign neoplastic change in a pre-existing naevus sebaceous (organoid naevus). Thus, most occur on the scalp. Occurrence of syringocystadenoma is marked by the development of a nodule which grows steadily and may ulcerate to produce an irregular crusty patch (a). Syringocystadenoma papilliferum arising de novo may occur on the face or elsewhere and presents as a single or several papules in childhood which enlarge and develop an irregular warty crusting surface around puberty.

The tumour is a cystic cavity lined by a papillary epithelial proliferation (b) which, if it has opened onto the skin surface, produces the red friable appearance of the lesion seen clinically. The lining epithelium (c) is double layered with an inner layer of columnar eosinophilic cells representing apocrine secretory cells, and an outer layer of cuboidal, small, darkly staining cells. There is frequently a lymphocyte and plasma cell infiltration of the stroma of the lesion (c), but early lesions often lack the inflammatory component. Apocrine glands are frequently seen in the dermis around the lesion and connect with the larger cystic areas.

Hidradenoma papilliferum is a very similar tumour found only in women and is confined to the labia majora and perineum. They are small, flesh-coloured, intra-dermal nodules. Histologically, the lesion consists of a nodule in the dermis, surrounded by a pseudocapsule of compressed dermal fibrous tissue. The nodule is composed of papillary fronds and cystic spaces lined by a double layer of cells. The inner layer is columnar and cuboidal with eosinophilic cytoplasm and apocrine characteristics (see Fig. 3.13). The outer cell layer is made up of smaller, darkly staining cells with characteristics of myoepithelial cells.

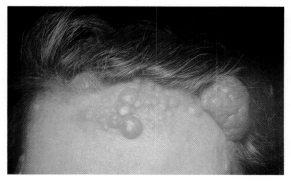

(a)

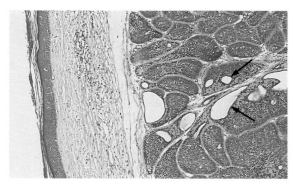

(b)

Fig. 20.20(a) & (b). Cylindroma

These lesions may be either solitary or multiple. Solitary lesions develop in early adult life on the face and scalp as in (a), and gradually increase in size. Multiple cylindromas show autosomal dominant inheritance and also occur most commonly on the scalp and face. They first appear early in adult life and increase in both size and number with the passage of time, so that by middle-age the scalp may be almost replaced by large numbers of tumours that are discrete, telangiectatic, smooth-surfaced, round, skin-coloured or pinkish, and of varying sizes. They may be associated with multiple trichoepitheliomas.

They consist of multiple, sharply demarcated islands of cells, each surrounded by a well-defined, hyaline, pink-staining sheath of basal lamina-like material. The cell islands fit together in close apposition with scant collagen stroma in between. At high magnification, the islands contain two cell types; small darkly staining cells (major component), and smaller numbers of paler, larger cells. Occasionally ductal lumina lined by two cell layers are seen within the islands (arrowed).

Malignant skin appendage tumours

Three types of malignant skin appendage tumour are commonly recognized, although all are rare.

1. **Carcinoma of sebaceous glands** usually occurs on the eyelids, face and scalp as a nodule rather like a basal cell carcinoma. They are characterized by aggressive local behaviour and are composed of lobulated nests of pleomorphic cells showing sebaceous differentiation.

2. **Eccrine carcinomas** may histologically resemble adenocarcinoma of the breast which is not surprising considering the origin of the breast from modified sweat glands. Ductal eccrine carcinoma shows neoplastic ductal structures lined by atypical epithelial cells infiltrating the dermis. Mucoid carcinoma is characterized by lakes of mucin surrounding small nests and acini of carcinoma cells. Adenoid-cystic carcinoma of eccrine origin has been described.

Because of the close resemblance to primary carcinoma of breast, metastatic mammary carcinoma should be considered before a diagnosis of primary eccrine carcinoma is made.

3. **Apocrine carcinoma** occurs in the axillae, perineum and scalp, and shows the pattern of an adenocarcinoma in which gland lumina are lined by atypical apocrine cells.

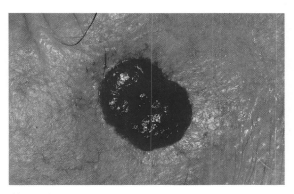

(a)

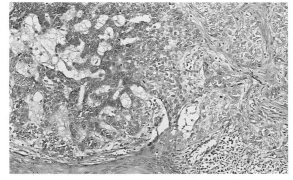

(b)

Fig. 20.21(a) & (b). Malignant skin appendage tumour

This is an eccrine carcinoma from the skin of the anterior chest, near the axilla, of an elderly man. It presented as a raised irregular red nodule which rapidly ulcerated. Histologically, note the architectural and cytological atypia of the glandular epithelium.

21.   Vascular malformations and tumours

Introduction

Skin lesions due to abnormal blood vessels are common, and many of the clinical manifestations of inflammatory skin disease are the result of transient disorder of structure and function of dermal blood vessels (e.g. erythema, urtication, purpura). Of the non-transient skin lesions due to persistently abnormal blood vessels, most are probably developmental malformations (hamartomas) and very few are true neoplasms. A typical example of a hamartomatous vascular malformation is the 'portwine stain' (flat haemangioma, naevus telangiectaticus). This common abnormality is nearly always present at birth as a flat, uniformly coloured, puplish-red or pink area of well-demarcated discoloration, often on the face, neck or limb. It may be faint or deeply coloured and extensive. The appearance is due to enormously dilated dermal blood vessels which are lined with rather flat endothelial cells; there is no vascular proliferation. Very red lesions, with large numbers of vessels, are treatable with the Argon laser because light of this frequency is absorbed by red cells with subsequent thrombosis and disintegration of vessels.

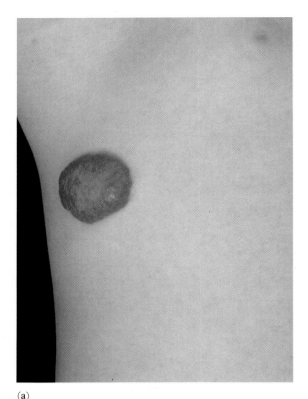

(a)

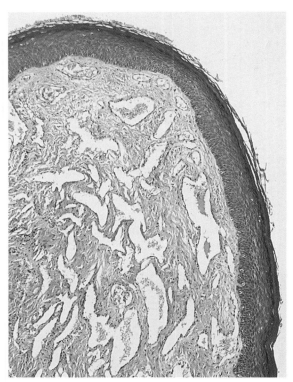

(b)

Fig. 21.1(a) & (b). Strawberry naevus (capillary haemangioma)

This is another very common vascular lesion. They are frequent on the buttocks and face, but are not present at birth; they appear after two to six months and grow quickly, usually to 2–4 cm in diameter. They are firm, rubbery, mottled red-pink tumours which protrude from, rather than grow in, the skin (a) and often ulcerate. The appearances are due to masses of proliferating endothelial cells and vascular

channels (b). Mitoses may be prominent. Lesions always shrink, usually after 12 to 24 months, and the structure is gradually replaced by collagen to leave a boggy white scar. However, there may be much deeper rubbery purple lesions beneath strawberry naevi; these are called cavernous haemangiomas and rarely regress. These are much more substantial because they consist of masses of endothelial-lined dermal vessels embedded in a matrix of collagen and fibroblasts.

Fig. 21.2(a), (b) & (c). Pyogenic granuloma

Another very common lesion, that usually appears suddenly as a rapidly enlarging, bright red, 0.5–2 cm cherry-like nodule (a). They bleed easily on contact and are usually found on the face and hands but can occur anywhere: children and adults are affected.

   Histologically they are composed of a proliferating mass of mainly small blood vessels (arrowed in (b), embedded in an oedematous stroma, and raised as a nodule above the level of the surrounding normal skin. There is usually a prominent large vessel at the depths of the lesion. A distinct feature is a waisted 'collaretate' of slightly thickened epidermis at its periphery (b). The epidermis over the surface of the lesion is stretched thin and almost invariably ulcerates; by the time the lesions are excised there is usually an acute inflammatory exudate and slough on the surface, and a heavy neutrophil infiltrate in the stroma of the lesion. This, and the collarette are useful distinguishing features from capillary haemangioma with which it can be confused histologically. Occasionally, satellite lesions occur (c); removal of the lesion by curettage with diathermy of the artery at the base is effective treatment. Despite their histological similarities to haemangiomas, these are acquired lesions rather than development abnormalities, and often follow an episode of trauma.

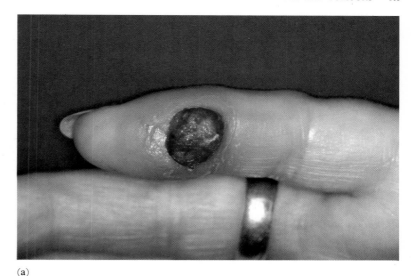

(a)

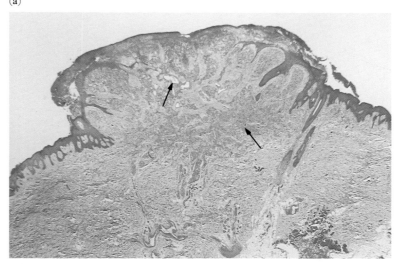

(b)

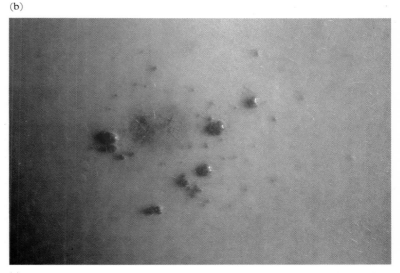

(c)

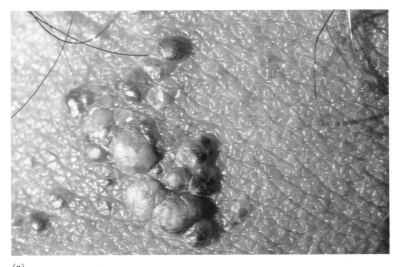

(a)

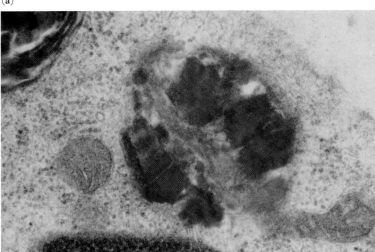

(b)

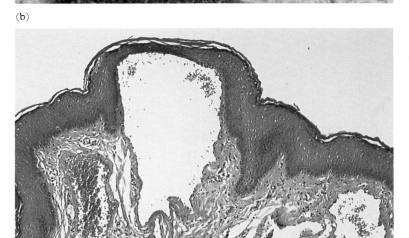

(c)

Fig. 21.3(a), (b) & (c).
Angiokeratoma

These are punctate protruding vascular lesions, usually 1–10 mm in diameter (a), which blanch easily with pressure. Their main significance is that they occur in Fabry's disease, both in affected males and in female hemizygotes, and are widespread, being greatest in number on the scrotum, trunk and limbs. The disease is a result of lysosomal α-galactosidase deficiency which results in intracellular accumulation of glycolipid in vascular smooth muscle and endothelium. Renal, cardiac and cerebrovascular involvement leads to death in the 40s and 50s. The diagnosis is confirmed by electron microscopy of vascular endothelium which reveals the characteristic dense laminated lysosomal inclusions (arrows in (b)), and by finding extremely low levels of α-galactosidase A. Rarer disorders, such as those of glycoprotein degradation, are also associated with widespread angiokeratomas. Localized angiokeratomas are clinically and histologically identical but are usually found on the fingers and toes (Mibelli) or scrotum (Fordyce); occasionally, larger lesions occur on the trunk. The histological features of angiokeratoma are simply greatly dilated upper dermal capillaries (c); the associated epidermal changes are very variable, from trivial acanthosis to dense hyperkeratosis and parakeratosis.

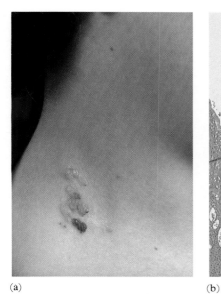

(a)

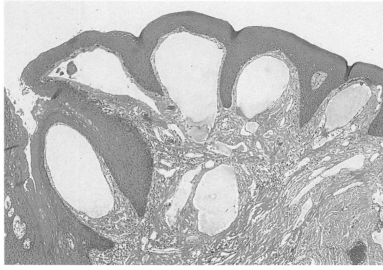

(b)

Fig. 21.4(a) & (b). Lymphangioma

These may be superficial or deep. Superficial lesions usually become apparent in childhood and frequently enlarge slowly. They appear as 'frog spawn' on the skin, a collection of superficial transparent fluid-filled blebs, each 1–5 mm in diameter (lymphangioma circumscriptum). Sometimes the fluid is blood-stained (a), and the lesion obscured by overlying hyperkeratosis. They are common on the trunk and thighs. As expected, the histology shows dilated endothelial-lined lymphatic vessels close to the surface with a thin covering of epidermis, as in (b); this is why patients frequently complain that the lesions weep. Although they

look superficial, they arise from abnormal, deep, cistern-like subcutaneous lymphatics, and surgical removal of the visible portion invariably results in recurrence and cosmetic deterioration. Deep (cavernous) lymphangiomas are much less common and present as soft, compressible, sometimes painful, subcutaneous masses, often on limbs. Similarly, they consist of dilated masses of lymphatics but in a collagen matrix. Cystic hygroma is a soft tissue lymphangiomatous hamartoma, usually in the neck, resulting from dilatation of the disordered lymphatic component of a mixed connective tissue hamartoma in which abnormal adipose tissue, blood vessels and nerves can also be found.

NEOPLASMS OF BLOOD VESSELS

Fig. 21.5(a) & (b). Glomus tumour

These uncommon lesions present as single, often very tender, compressible, flesh-coloured or bluish nodules about 0.5 cm in diameter, often on the distal part of a limb or under a nail (a). There may be sudden episodes of pain and a lesion may be difficult to spot. Glomus tumours originate from temperature-regulating arteriovenous shunts in the lower dermis. They are composed of narrow, branching, vascular channels lined internally by flattened endothelium and cuffed by layers of compact glomus cells (b). There is a collagenous fibrous capsule which may contain mast cells. Leiomyomas can be distinguished because they are red, solid and occur proximally; eccrine spiradenomas may be difficult to distinguish clinically.

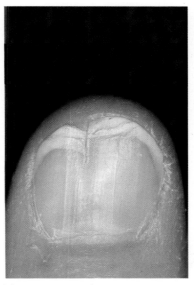

(a)

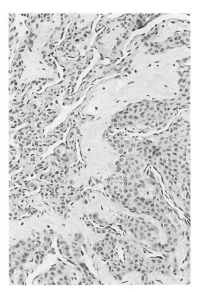

(b)

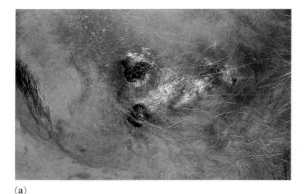

(a)

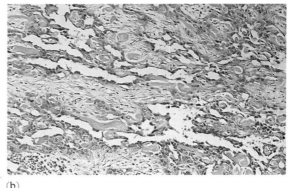

(b)

Fig. 21.6(a) & (b). Angiosarcoma of skin

Angiosarcoma involving the skin almost always occurs in the face or scalp of elderly people. It may start as a flat area of erythema but may be more intensely coloured and resemble an irregular bruise. The lesions expand irregularly and may develop nodules, haemorrhage and ulceration. The malignant infiltration always extends beyond the visible discoloured margins of the lesion, even as far as the trunk, rendering adequate surgical excision difficult; spread to local lymph nodes is common. Angiosarcoma may supervene in chronic lymphoedema of the arm following radical axillary lymph node clearance for carcinoma of the breast (Stewart-Treves syndrome). It occurs very rarely in portwine stains.

Histologically, the tumour is ill-defined and mainly occupies the dermis but often extends into subcutis. It is composed of irregular connecting vascular channels (b) lined by endothelial cells which show the cytological features suggestive of malignancy; they are large, and show nuclear and cytoplasmic pleomorphism, with increased mitotic activity. The degree of differentiation of the tumour varies from site to site, with the better differentiated areas usually at the periphery, which is the usual site of biopsy; care must therefore be exercised in the interpretation of histology from such biopsies because of the danger of understating the degree of malignancy.

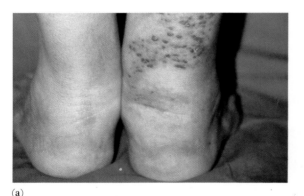

(a)

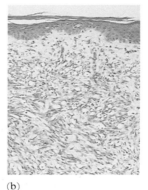

(b)

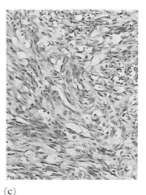

(c)

Fig. 21.7(a), (b) & (c). Kaposi's sarcoma

There has been a striking change in the epidemiology of this disease in the USA and Europe, due largely to AIDS with which it is closely associated. Not only is it commoner but the disease has changed character. Classical (European and American) Kaposi's sarcoma is a slowly progressive disorder of the elderly, especially men, resulting in gradually increasing numbers of purplish papules and nodules usually on the legs (a). Metastasis to lymph nodes and viscera is uncommon. Kaposi's sarcoma in Central and East Africa is much more aggressive, occurring in children and young adults with rapid spread, resulting in death. AIDS-related Kaposi mimics this pattern to some extent as it occurs in the 20s and 30s and is usually widespread, especially in lymph nodes and the gastrointestinal tract; the lesions may not involve the skin at all. Skin lesions occur most frequently on the trunk and head as firm rubbery oval macules or papules which frequently enlarge into nodules and plaques. They are usually pink or red and may become tinged with brown due to melanin. Mucosal lesions (palate, oropharynx) are also frequent.

Histologically, the established lesions have two components, an irregular system of proliferating vascular channels lined by endothelial cells which are prominent but show little pleomorphism or nuclear atypia (cf. angiosarcoma: Fig. 21.6), and a spindle-celled fibrous component often traversed by narrow vascular channels with flat endothelium. Depending on the age of the lesion, there may be an interstitial infiltrate of chronic inflammatory cells (early lesions) and oedematous collagen containing haemosiderin (later lesions).

22. Lymphoma and prelymphoma in skin

Introduction

Infiltration of the upper dermis by lymphoid cells is a very common finding in a wide range of inflammatory and reactive skin diseases, but their cytological features and their distribution (around dermal vessels and skin appendages) usually indicates that they are part of an inflammatory or immunological reaction. Lymphocytes may also encroach upon epithelial structures such as epidermis (exocytosis) and pilosebaceous units as part of certain types of inflammatory skin disease, although this infiltration does not imply malignancy. Malignant lymphoma does occur in the skin, and the clinical and histological distinction between this and a non-neoplastic heavy lymphocytic infiltrate is one of the most difficult areas in diagnostic dermatopathology. Furthermore, there are a number of skin conditions which are believed to predispose to the eventual development of malignant lymphoma, but there is inadequate information about their natural history to quantify the risk.

In a book of this type it is not possible to explore the complexities of the problem, particularly since, as in other areas of lymphoma pathology, our understanding of certain aspects of the pathogenesis and diagnosis of the conditions is proceeding rapidly. This is partly due to the use of immunocytochemical techniques to identify subsets of B and T lymphocytes and other accessory cells in the lympho-reticular system (see Fig. 22.13).

The conditions to be dealt with here can be considered under the following headings:
1. True malignant lymphoma in the skin;
2. Conditions which may be precursors of lymphoma;
3. Conditions which mimic lymphoma clinically and/or histologically.

MALIGNANT LYMPHOMA OF SKIN

Any type of malignant lymphoma may involve the skin when the disease is generalized (Stage IV); such cases are rarely a diagnostic problem since the previous history is usually clear, but biopsy is helpful for confirmation and to exclude other skin disorders. The types of malignant haemopoietic neoplasms which most commonly involve skin secondarily are leukaemias and non-Hodgkin's lymphoma. Hodgkin's disease rarely presents as a skin lesion, and it is unlikely that it ever originates in skin. Skin lesions are uncommon during the course of the disease; they consist of pink-red papules or nodules, often grouped. The leukaemias which most commonly involve the skin are chronic lymphocytic leukaemia and the acute monoblastic and myelomonoblastic leukaemias.

Cutaneous B cell lymphoma

This is discussed in Fig. 22.3.

Cutaneous T cell lymphoma

For the dermatologist, the most important type of lymphoma is that which probably originates in the skin and is a malignant proliferation of T lymphocytes. This group of disorders has been officially designated cutaneous T cell lymphoma (CTCL) and encompasses the conditions formerly known as mycosis fungoides and Sézary syndrome.

Mycosis fungoides usually evolves from small to large plaques, nodules then tumours. The patterns are discussed in detail in Figures 22.1 and 22.2. In recent studies, disseminated disease occurs in about half the cases.

Accurate diagnosis of cutaneous T cell lymphoma depends on the correct identification of malignant T lymphocytes.

The malignant T cell and its recognition

T lymphocytes are thymus-derived lymphocytes responsible for cellular immunity. Malignant T cells are generally large cells (approximately 20–30 μm in diameter) with an irregular cerebriform nucleus with dense but marginated nuclear chromatin which gives the appearance of a hyperchromatic cell by light microscopy. Smaller cells (less than 12 μm in diameter) with convoluted nuclei which are less hyperchromatic can be found in a number of reactive inflammatory skin conditions, especially severe dermatitis, and are probably not malignant. However, size alone is not always a reliable criterion and should be considered in conjunction with nuclear changes. The histological diagnosis of cutaneous T cell lymphoma is based on the demonstration of malignant T cells within the skin (or in blood, bone marrow or lymph node in Sézary syndrome). In the plaque and tumour stages, malignant T cells are usually abundant and are the predominant cell infiltrating dermis and epidermis. The histological diagnosis of cutaneous T cell lymphoma using only routine H & E-stained paraffin sections can be difficult, particularly in the early plaque stage; fortunately modern laboratory techniques are making the task easier:

1. **Thin (1–2 μm) resin sections** allow high resolution light microscopy, thus permitting more accurate identification of malignant T cells with their characteristic large size and convoluted nuclei.

2. **Electron microscopy**: the appearance of an undoubted malignant T cell is characteristic (see Fig. 22.1(d)).

3. **Immunocytochemical methods** allow lymphocytes to be classified into B and T types using B and T cell markers. Furthermore, T cells can be divided into 'helper' and 'suppressor' subsets using immunocytochemical methods. In cutaneous T cell lymphoma, the malignant T cells are mainly T helper cells.

4. **Langerhans cell changes**: Langerhans cells are normally present in both epidermis and dermis, but in CTCL they are found in increased numbers in both sites, usually in close association with the malignant T cells. The presence of increased numbers of Langerhans cells in the dermis is a particularly valuable indication of T cell lymphoma in skin lesions in the erythematous patch stage when malignant T cells may be scanty. Langerhans cells can be identified either ultrastructurally (see Fig. 3.8) or immunocytochemically (Langerhans cells show T6 [CD 1] positivity).

From the above, it is apparent that accurate histological diagnosis in cases of suspected cutaneous T cell lymphoma requires close co-operation between dermatologist and pathologist. Biopsies from several sites are necessary; the skin sample should be sent fresh and unfixed to the laboratory as soon as possible after biopsy so that part can be snap-frozen and cryostat sections prepared for the immunocytochemical staining for T cell subsets and Langerhans cells. Samples from the remaining tissue can be processed for electron microscopy and resin sections for high resolution light microscopy. Increasing use of techniques such as these should improve the accuracy of diagnosis in this group of disorders.

Fig. 22.1(a)–(e). Cutaneous T cell Lymphoma: patch and plaque stages (*illustrations opposite*)
Clinically, the lesions are either small, erythematous, well-defined pinkish-red patches or small plaques with a wrinkled scaly surface (a), or more raised, large plaques (b), or a combination of the two. They often first appear on the trunk as patches which are fixed and slowly enlarge into raised plaques. In the patch and small plaque stages there is an unimpressive mixed inflammatory cell infiltrate, composed of lymphocytes and histiocytes, situated in the upper dermis, particularly the papillary dermis. There is always some degree of infiltration of the epidermis by lymphocytes (epidermotropism) without significant associated spongiosis, but spongiosis may be seen where the epidermal infiltrate is heavy and the lesion is clinically scaly, usually when the lesions are at the large plaque stage (c). The lymphocytes may be scattered singly in the epidermis, or may aggregate into small clusters (Pautrier microabscesses). High resolution light microscopy, for example, using thin resin sections as in (e), shows that the infiltrating lymphocytes are large and have cerebriform nuclei, indicating that they are malignant T lymphocytes. Sometimes the epidermis shows irregular lengthening of the rete ridges and the papillae are oedematous, containing only a few lymphoid cells which mainly lie deeper in the subpapillary dermis; this pattern may clinically resemble a psoriasiform dermatitis. Electron microscopical examination of the cell population infiltrating the epidermis and dermis will reveal that a proportion of the 'lymphocytoid' cells are in fact proliferating Langerhans cells and that the true lymphocytes present have the ultrastructural features of malignant T lymphocytes viz large size and complex cerebriform nucleus (d). Immunocytochemical methods using T6 (CD 1) as a Langerhans cell marker and T4 (CD 4) as a T helper cell marker reveals the same, but provides the additional information that the majority of T cells are T helper cells. These subtle changes are not usually discernible in a routine paraffin section, and it is rarely possible to confidently confirm or deny a diagnosis of CTCL at the erythematous patch stage unless special laboratory methods are used. At the plaque stage the diagnosis is usually more easily made histologically, although it is always advisable to use immunocytochemistry and electron microscopy for confirmation, since similar excesses of epidermal and dermal T lymphocytes and Langerhans cells can be seen in the inflammatory skin reaction in some patterns of chronic contact dermatitis although the T cells are smaller, less hyperchromatic and have less convoluted nuclei. By light microscopy, a useful differentiator is that in many inflammatory skin conditions mast cells and basophils are numerous in the dermal infiltrate, but are scanty in CTCL.

By the time the plaques are large and raised, the infiltrate in the upper dermis is heavier and contains a much higher proportion of malignant T cells. Similarly, the epidermal infiltrate is more marked, with malignant T cells and Langerhans cells scattered in the somewhat thickened epidermis and Pautrier microabscesses may be larger and more numerous.

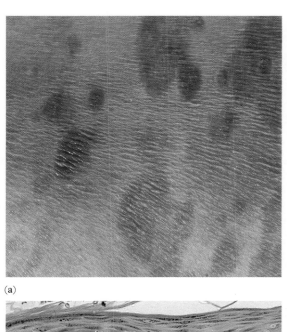

(a)

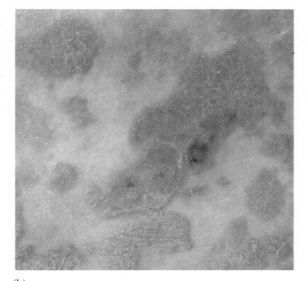

(b)

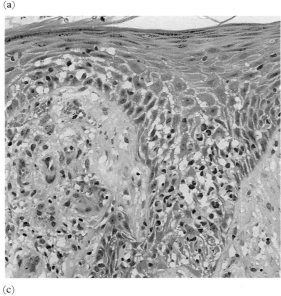

(c)

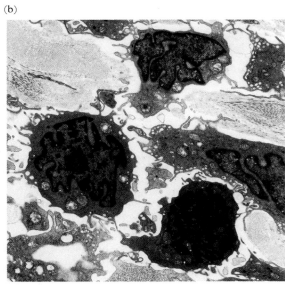

(d)

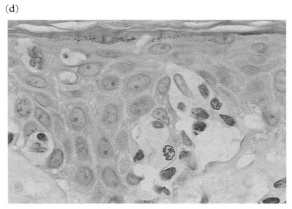

(e)

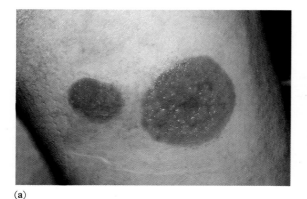

(a)

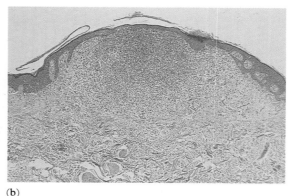

(b)

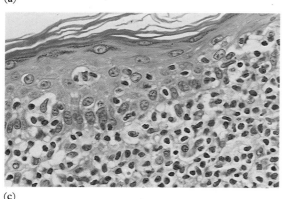

(c)

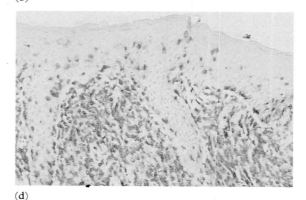

(d)

Fig. 22.2(a)–(e). Cutaneous T cell Lymphoma: tumour stage

At the tumour stage there are raised red nodules (a), usually arising on a background of plaques and patches. The tumours increase in size, often with central ulceration. Rarely they arise de novo without pre-existing patch or plaque stages; this is more common in B cell lymphoma (see Fig. 22.3).

By the tumour stage there is little histological doubt about the diagnosis of lymphoma; the dermis is extensively infiltrated by malignant T cells which spread into subcutaneous fat and infiltrate and destroy skin appendages and the overlying epidermis, as seen in (b) and (c). Immunocytochemistry (T4) identifies the infiltrating cells as T cells (d).

In cases of the Sézary syndrome associated with T cell lymphoma in the skin, malignant T cells may be seen within the lumina of dermal blood vessels (arrow in (e)), as well as in the dermis and epidermis.

Sézary syndrome is defined as erythroderma, lymphadenopathy and more than 10% atypical lymphocytes in peripheral blood. The morphological characteristics of these Sézary cells are convoluted (cerebriform) hyperchromatic nuclei in a lymphocyte greater than 15 μm in diameter, i.e. they are like the cells infiltrating the skin in CTCL. Most patients with Sézary syndrome do not have

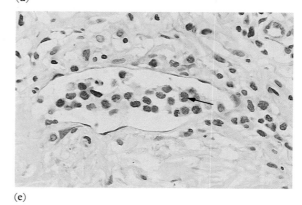

(e)

the skin lesions typical of mycosis fungoides but the abnormal cells are present in the skin. Probably less than half of patients with the clinical features of the Sézary syndrome have CTCL, and the histological distinction between neoplastic and non-neoplastic disease is based on attempts to differentiate between malignant and benign atypical T cells in the infiltrating and circulating lymphocyte population.

Fig. 22.3(a), (b) & (c). Cutaneous B cell lymphoma

Clinically, the lesions usually appear as a mixture of red nodules coalescing into plaques, or an isolated red, often oval, plaque (a).

Histologically, there is a diffuse infiltrate by lymphoid cells; note the lack of follicle formation, the sparing of the dermis immediately beneath the epidermal basement membrane, and the extension of the infiltrate into the subcutaneous fat (b). Micrograph (c) shows the cytological detail of the lymphoma; note that the cells show the characteristics of B lymphocytes, with rounded nuclei showing none of the cerebriform pattern seen in T lymphocytes. There is moderate pleomorphism, with some large nucleolated forms. Compare the pattern of infiltration in this picture with that of benign lymphocytoma cutis (Fig. 22.9) and Jessner's benign lymphocytic infiltrate (Fig. 22.10), both of which can be confused with cutaneous B cell lymphoma.

Even when the disease presents with cutaneous lesions, the vast majority show evidence of concurrent systemic involvement on examination and investigation, and the remainder develop disseminated disease within the next 1 or 2 years. Any of the types of B cell lymphoma which occur elsewhere can occur in the skin, but the types which most commonly involve skin are follicle centre cell lymphomas, lymphoplasma cytoid lymphoma and immunoblastic lymphoma. Accurate identification of the nature of the B cell lymphoma depends on the cytological and immunocytochemical features of the cells. (see Table 22.1, p.183)

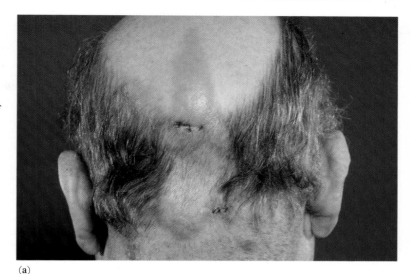

(a)

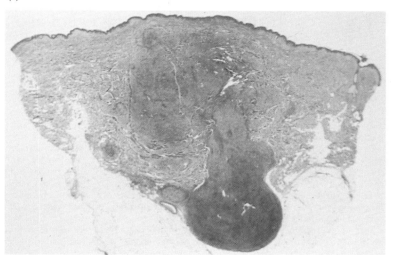

(b)

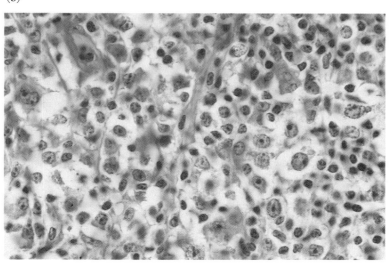

(c)

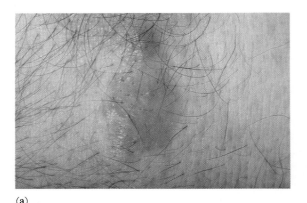

(a)

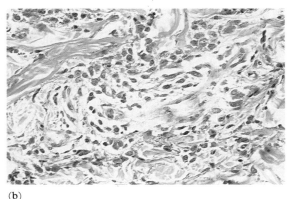

(b)

Fig. 22.4(a) & (b). Leukaemic infiltrate in skin
This is uncommon and usually manifests as flesh-coloured
or pink papules or nodules (a) on the trunk in association
with chronic lymphocytic leukaemia or monocytic
leukaemia.

Histologically, there is an accumulation of primitive
blast cells in the dermis, mainly around dermal vessels (b).
Chloroacetate esterase methods suggested that the primitive
leukaemic cells had a myeloid origin. The patient had acute
myelomonocytic (M4) leukaemia.

CONDITIONS WHICH MAY BE PRECURSORS OF LYMPHOMAS
(PRE-MYCOTIC ERUPTIONS)

Some skin conditions are considered to be precursors of cutaneous T cell lymphoma, but it must be emphasized
that the risk of development of lymphoma in an individual with one of these premycotic eruptions is not always
clear. Regular follow-up, with repeated biopsies, is essential to define their natural history.

**Fig. 22.5(a) & (b) (resin) (c) & (d). Fixed scaly
eruptions** (*illustrations opposite*)
These were formerly grouped together under the name
parapsoriasis en plaque, but two patterns are now
recognized. One of these eventually proceeds to lymphoma,
while the other pattern is termed *chronic superficial scaly
dermatitis* or digitate dermatitis (equivalent to parapsoriasis
en plaque—small plaque type) and has a characteristically
symmetrical distribution of persistent round, oval or
finger-like red patches with slight scaling, as in (a). The
redness is a result of prominence of upper dermal blood
vessels and a scanty infiltrate of lymphocytes in upper
dermis, mainly around blood vessels; this infiltrate is
neither dense nor thick and hence the plaques are flat rather
than raised. Some lymphoid cells are also found scattered in
the epidermis, sometimes associated with mild spongiosis,
which produces the parakeratosis responsible for the fine
surface scale (b).

The fixed scaly eruption which may be a precursor of
cutaneous T cell lymphoma closely resembles the patch and
early plaque stages of mycosis fungoides; see Figures 22.1(a)
and (b). The lesions are widespread but asymmetrical;

initially flat and pink, they become slightly raised and
redder with time, and acquire a wrinkled scaly suface (c)
sometimes resembling plaques of psoriasis. This pattern
was formerly known as parapsoriasis en plaque—large
plaque type and should be regarded as a pre-CTCL lesion.
Compared with the chronic superficial scaly dermatitis
lesion, this shows a much denser lymphoid infiltrate in
upper dermis (d), hence the greater redness and raised
nature of the lesion. The degree of scaliness is directly
proportional to the degree of lymphocytic infiltration into
the epidermis (epidermotropism: see Fig. 4.9(b)) and is
usually greater than in chronic superficial scaly dermatitis.

Immunocytochemical methods show that a proportion
of the lymphoid cells in dermis and epidermis in the fixed
scaly eruptions are T cells, being more numerous in the
large-plaque parapsoriasis type. Although these two lesions
can usually be distinguished clinically, it may be difficult
histologically since the distinction is largely a matter of
degree. It can be even more difficult to differentiate
histologically between large plaque parapsoriasis and
mycosis fungoides without recourse to electron microscopy
and immunocytochemistry.

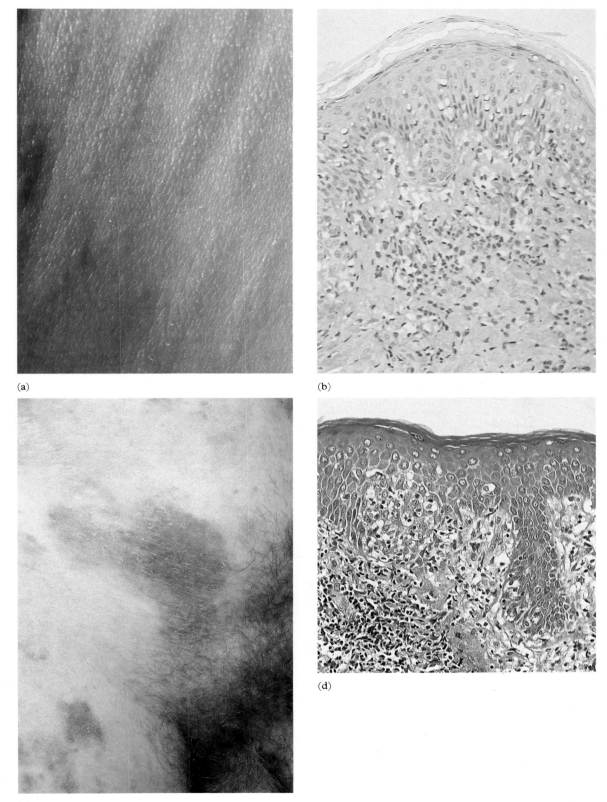

(a)

(b)

(c)

(d)

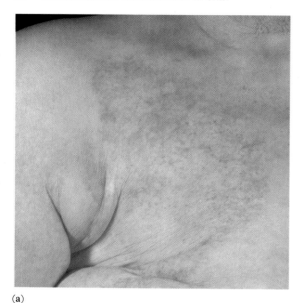

(a)

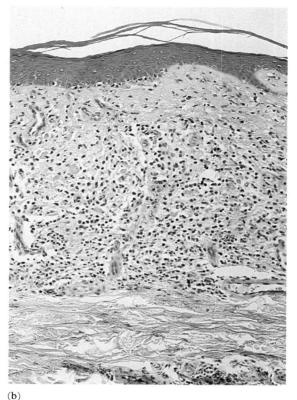

(b)

Fig. 22.6(a), (b) & (c). Poikiloderma

Poikiloderma is skin atrophy with telangiectasia and
reticulate hyperpigmentation (a). It may be widespread, or
present as localized patches. The histological changes are an
upper dermal infiltrate of lymphoid cells and histiocytes
which extend up diffusely into the lower layers of the
epidermis where they disrupt the basal layer. The epidermis
is atrophic but with overlying hyperkeratosis; prominent
dilated upper dermal vessels are present here and there
amongst the lymphoid infiltrate (b). Long-standing lesions
are marked by increased numbers of dermal pigment-laden
macrophages, the result of chronic basal cell damage and
melanin release into the underlying dermis. The nature of
the lymphoid infiltrate is important; the presence of a high
proportion of atypical large lymphoid cells, with the nuclear
configuration of T cells (arrowed in (c)), suggests that the
poikilodermatous rash is an early manifestation of cutaneous
T cell lymphoma (c). Plaques and tumorous nodules of
mycosis fungoides may co-exist with poikilodermatous
patches.

    Poikilodermatous lesions may also occur in association
with dermatomyositis and lupus erythematosus, in which
the characteristic clinical appearances are the result of
inflammatory cell destruction of the basal cell layer with
associated upper dermal vascular dilatation. It can also be
seen in association with syndromes such as dyskeratosis
congenita and in some drug reactions.

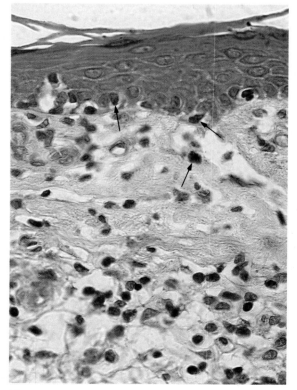

(c)

Fig. 22.7. Follicular mucinosis

This manifests as well-defined red infiltrated, rather translucent, papules and plaques, usually spreading up the sides of the face; when it involves hair-bearing skin, alopecia is usual. In a few cases the lesions are larger and extend beyond the face and neck; it is this variant which may indicate developing cutaneous T cell lymphoma, and more characteristic plaques and tumours of the mycosis fungoides type may co-exist.

Histologically, there is a mixed chronic inflammatory cell infiltrate, comprising lymphocytes and histiocytes with a few plasma cells and eosinophils, in the dermis, particularly concentrated around the pilosebaceous apparatus, affected units of which show characteristic vacuolar and mucinous degeneration (arrows), in which abundant acid mucopoly-saccharides can be demonstrated with the Alcian Blue stain. In the type associated with lymphoma, the cellular infiltrate is suggestive of lymphoma, with a high proportion of large, atypical T lymphocytes.

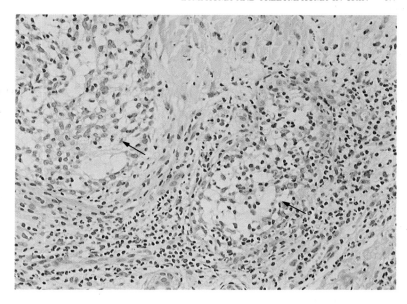

In addition to the above, there are two conditions which show some histological similarities to cutaneous lymphoma, but in which progression to lymphoma is unusual. These are *lymphomatoid papulosis* and *lymphomatoid granulomatosis*.

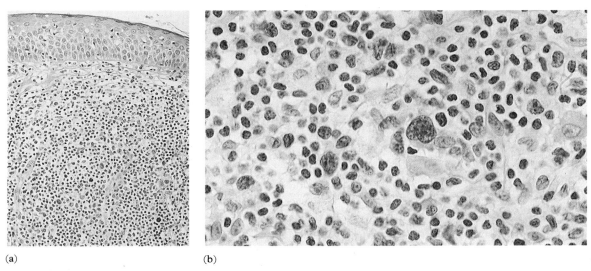

(a)   (b)

Fig. 22.8(a) & (b). Lymphomatoid papulosis

This presents as recurrent episodes of papules, mainly on the back, which ulcerate and heal over several weeks to leave a scar. It usually occurs in adults aged 30–60, most commonly in men in their 50s. Each papule is initially oedematous, dome-shaped and reddish-brown in colour, often with a shiny surface. The disease may persist for a few months to many years.

The lesions show a heavy infiltrate of histiocytic and lymphoid cells in the upper dermis (b), usually associated with marked oedema of the papillary dermis and infiltration

of the thinned epidermis by identical cells. Many of the lymphoid cells show nuclear and cytoplasmic pleomorphism and mitoses can be numerous; the appearances of these cells suggest that they are malignant lymphoid blast cells (b). Immunocytochemical studies have shown that these abnormal cells are T lymphocytes. Blood vessels in the centre of the infiltrate often show endothelial swelling and some degree of vessel wall oedema and inflammation. Despite the 'malignant' histological features, the disease usually runs a benign course, although the development of malignant lymphoma has been reported.

Lymphomatoid granulomatosis is a rare systemic disease in which cutaneous manifestations are common, and may be the presenting symptom. The disorder has been regarded as an example of systemic lymphocytic vasculitis since that is the lesion which is most prominent in the lung parenchyma, the other major organ involved; however, current concepts hold that it is probably an unusual pattern of T cell lymphoma. Careful histological examination of the skin lesions usually reveals a lymphocytic vasculitis component, although the vessel involvement may be obscured by the heavy infiltrate of lymphocytes, histiocytes and plasma cells present. The vasculitic component of the lesion is best seen at its edges where the cellular infiltrate is lightest, and the use of an elastic-van Gieson is often helpful; occasionally, foci of neutrophilic vasculitis can be found. Many of the lymphoid cells present are pleomorphic and atypical, a useful distinguishing feature from other types of cutaneous lymphocytic vasculitis (see Ch. 12).

The skin lesions present as raised red plaques or papules, the largest of which tend to ulcerate; they are often extensive and indolent.

Untreated, most patients die of progressive pulmonary involvement, but a proportion (probably 10%) develop a more typical clinical picture of systematized malignant lymphoma.

In all of the conditions which may predispose to lymphoma, at the onset of the lesions it is impossible to determine on clinical and histological grounds whether a particular case is likely to become lymphomatous or not, although a particularly heavy lymphocytic infiltrate in which large hyperchromatic lymphoid cells are present in both dermis and epidermis is thought to indicate likely progression to CTCL. Nevertheless, the evidence (albeit inadequate) indicates that the majority behave in an entirely benign manner. A rare disorder, known either as Pagetoid reticulosis or Woringer-Kolopp disease, illustrates the occasional lack of correlation between histological features of malignancy and subsequent behaviour. These usually solitary raised red scaly plaques often on the lower extremities, show apparent invasion of upper dermis and epidermis by abnormal hyperchromatic lymphoid cells having the cytological and ultrastructural features of malignant T cells; Langerhans cells are also present, as in CTCL. However, the lesions are benign, and widespread CTCL does not develop.

Although no satisfactory predictive criteria for risk of lymphoma exist at present, immunocytochemical techniques may supply answers to the problem in the future.

CONDITIONS WHICH MIMIC LYMPHOMA

Most skin lymphoma presents as raised red plaques or nodules, but a number of non-malignant inflammatory or reactive conditions can present in a similar way. Usually the distinction between benign and malignant raised red plaques is clear both clinically and histologically, but there are a number of lesions where histological distinction can be extremely difficult, usually because of either the heaviness of the lymphocytic infiltrate, or because of the presence of pleomorphic lymphocytoid cells with cytological features of malignancy. Some of the conditions which can mimic malignant lymphoma include:

1. **Drug reactions**: allergic reaction to drugs have replaced syphilis as the great dermatological mimic (see Ch. 14) and certain drugs, such as Captopril, may produce lesions with clinical and histological features suggesting skin lymphoma. The history of drug ingestion and the resolution of the lesion after cessation of therapy indicates the true diagnosis.

2. **Reactions to insect bites and infestations such as scabies**: these may produce a very pleomorphic infiltrate of lymphocytes and other cells in the dermis and subcutis, some of the cells having cytological features suggesting malignancy.

3. **Reactions to virus infection**: usually herpes. The development of raised red plaques or nodules in resolving herpes lesions, e.g. shingles, can mimic lymphoma clinically, although histologically the lymphoid infiltrate is not usually frightening.

4. **Other local reactions**: occasional persistent local reactions to antigen may mimic lymphoma. The most common examples are at the site of tattoos and vaccinations.

5. **Lymphocytoma cutis**: see Figure 22.9.

6. **Jessner's lymphocytic infiltrate**: see Figure 22.10.

7. **Actinic reticuloid**: see Figure 22.11.

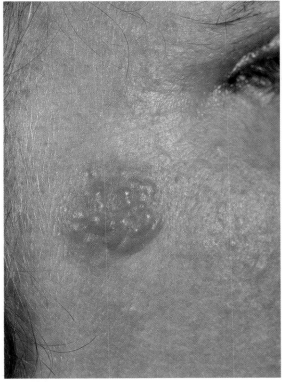

(a)

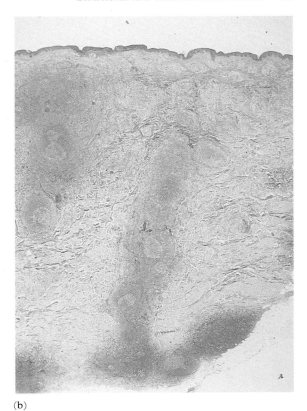

(b)

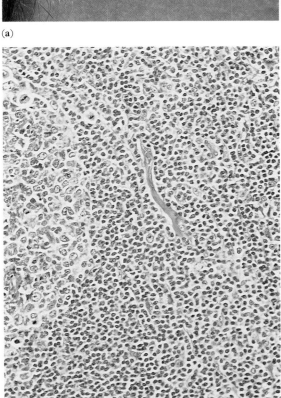

(c)

Fig. 22.9(a), (b) & (c). Lymphocytoma cutis

These lesions can appear anywhere on the body but occur most commonly on the face and neck, and present as single or grouped red-purple papules which enlarge into nodules and plaques which tend to persist (a). They are well-demarcated and have a normal, occasionally shiny epidermal covering. Occasionally a diffuse infiltrative form occurs. Histologically, the dermis shows large, rounded aggregates of lymphoid cells in upper and mid-dermis, sometimes extending into lower dermis particularly around skin appendages (b). The infiltrate is of small, mature B lymphocytes and larger lymphoid cells, with some macrophages and eosinophils. Varying degrees of lymphoid follicle formation can be seen in some of the larger aggregates (c). Blood vessels in the vicinity of the infiltrate are frequently thick-walled and show endothelial cell swelling. The roundness of the lymphoid aggregate is frequently less well defined at the upper border and the infiltrate of cells scatters diffusely into the papillary dermis though usually stops short of the dermo-epidermal junction, often leaving a narrow clear (Grenz) zone immediately beneath the epidermal basal lamina. Occasionally, a variant occurs in which the predominant lymphocyte is a larger, paler, more pleomorphic cell which is probably of follicle centre cell origin. These tend to occupy the central area of the rounded aggregates, with a peripheral rim of smaller lymphocytes around them. This pattern, sometimes called 'large cell lymphocytoma' is clinically identical to lymphocytoma cutis and should be regarded as a variant rather than a distinct entity.

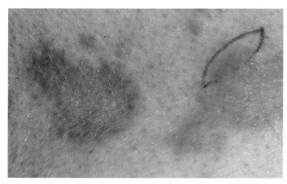

(a)

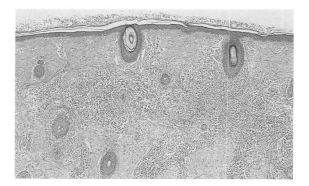

(b)

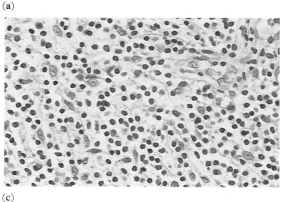

(c)

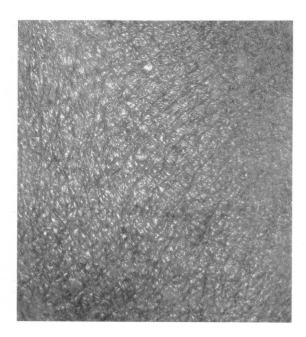

Fig. 22.10(a), (b) & (c). Jessner's lymphocytic infiltration

These are red papules and plaques (a) occuring most commonly on the face, but occasionally on the upper trunk. They progressively enlarge over 1–2 months then fade: this cycle often continues for several years. They are not usually fixed.

Histologically, this differs from lymphocytoma cutis in that the lymphocytic infiltrate (which may be dense) is largely confined to regions around blood vessels and skin appendages (b), and rarely rounds off to suggest attempts at follicle formation. Macrophages are less frequent and occasional plasma cells may be present. Although the accumulation is most marked in the dermis, lymphocytes may extend into subcutaneous fat around deep blood vessels and deep skin appendages. Solar and myxoid degeneration of dermal collagen (see Ch. 15) is a frequent associated finding. Because of its perivascular distribution, and the comparative uniformity of the lymphocyte type (c), this benign condition needs to be distinguished histologically from skin involvement in chronic lymphocytic leukaemia.

Fig. 22.11. Actinic reticuloid

This occurs in middle-aged or elderly men as severe persistent photosensitivity to UV and visible light. It is often due to persistent photocontact allergy to plant oleoresins. There is redness, oedema, induration and lichenification of light-exposed skin (a), initially on the face and neck, but often spreading to the trunk and covered sites.

There is a heavy infiltrate of mixed inflammatory cells in the upper and mid-dermis, often extending down into deep dermis, and even subcutis, mainly around blood vessels. The infiltrate consists of lymphocytes, histiocytes, with some plasma cells, eosinophils and occasional neutrophils; some of the lymphoid cells are large and atypical, suggesting lymphoma. The papillary dermis shows a mixture of cellular infiltrate and increased fibrosis, and some of the lymphoid cells may be present in the epidermis singly and in small clumps, thus mimicking CTCL. The upper dermal fibrosis is most marked in old, indurated lesions which clinically show significant lichenification, and such lesions also show the epidermal changes of a chronic traumatic dermatitis (lichen simplex chronicus: see Fig. 5.2); it is probable that these features are secondary to persistent rubbing or scratching. Despite the histological similarity to CTCL, the lesions improve if the patient is protected from light.

Histological distinction between benign and malignant lymphocytic proliferations

No single histological criterion can satisfactorily distinguish between benign and malignant B cell and T cell lymphocytic infiltrates of the skin, but a combination of features may point to the most likely diagnosis.

In general, malignant infiltrates are monomorphous and composed of medium to large lymphoid cells, whereas benign infiltrates contain small lymphocytes and are polymorphous, with a number of other cells present including histiocytes (often with phagocytosed nuclear debris). When large lymphocytic cells occur in benign infiltrates they are frequently well-demarcated from the small lymphocytes, often in a follicular or pseudofollicular pattern. Attempts at follicle production are common in benign lesions, whereas malignant infiltrates are usually diffuse, often extending into lower dermis and subcutis; benign lesions usually only extend into subcutaneous fat around blood vessels and skin appendages, except when caused by a deeply penetrating insect bite. Epidermal infiltration by lymphoid cells is common in malignant conditions, particularly T cell lymphomas, and CTCL is notable for the relative absence of spongiosis compared to the severity of the infiltrate; aggregations of lymphoid cells in the epidermis to form small clumps is highly suggestive of lymphoma. When, less commonly, lymphocytes infiltrate the epidermis in benign conditions, there is usually associated spongiosis and cell clumping is rare. High resolution light microscopy (e.g. thin 3 μm paraffin sections or 1–2 μm resin sections) usually enables the infiltrating lymphoid cells to be identified as B or T types (a T cell infiltrate is more likely to be lymphomatous than one composed largely of B cells).

Although these indicators may be useful, there remains an unsatisfactorily large proportion of cases in which the diagnosis is unclear; it is in this group that the future diagnostic use of immunocytochemistry provides hope of more accurate diagnosis. Table 22.1 summarizes some of the potentially valuable immunocytochemical reactions which may assist in the diagnosis of malignant lymphoma. Most methods can only be applied successfully to fresh frozen sections but immunoglobulins, and Pan-B/Pan-T cell markers of the CD45R group can be detected in paraffin sections.

Laboratory handling of suspected skin lymphoma specimens

To obtain the maximum information from such a skin biopsy, it is essential to have the facility to use all the available pathological techniques. These include immunocytochemistry, high resolution light microscopy and transmission electron microscopy. Since unfixed frozen sections are required for the most informative immunocytochemical methods (B and T subset markers), it is best if the biopsy is taken directly to the laboratory in a fresh, unfixed state, so that it can be divided into suitably sized and trimmed samples for frozen sections (for immunocytochemistry), embedding in an acrylic resin (for high resolution light microscopy) and embedding in an epoxy resin (for transmission electron microscopy). This is best done by prior arrangement.

Notes on other relevant conditions

Histiocytosis X

Despite its name, there is increasing evidence that this group of disorders is of Langerhans cell origin. Certainly in Letterer-Siwe disease, ultrastructural and immunocytochemical studies indicate that the predominant cell is a Langerhans-type cell. In the other two conditions included in the histiocytosis X group, Hand-Schüller-Christian disease and eosinophilic granuloma, similar cells are present, but are diluted by the presence of variable numbers of other cells, mainly lymphocytes, eosinophils and plasma cells. These latter two conditions mainly affect bones, and cutaneous manifestations are largely confined to the presentation as subcutaneous lumps originating in underlying bone, particularly in the skull. However, transitional forms occur, and skin lesions clinically like those in Letterer-Siwe disease can co-exist with osteolytic bony lesions, particularly in the Hand-Schüller-Christian variant.

Histiocytic proliferations

Histiocyte and macrophage accumulations in skin are a common feature of certain types of infection (e.g. leprosy: see Fig. 11.2) and reactive conditions (e.g. granuloma annulare: see Fig. 11.4). There remains a group of conditions, which are neither reactive nor lymphoma-related, in which histiocytic cells are an important component, e.g. xanthoma, xanthogranuloma, histiocytoma and its variants; some of these are discussed in Chapter 23.

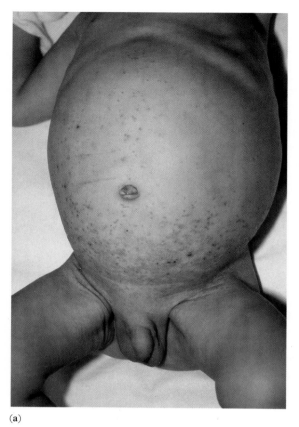

(a)

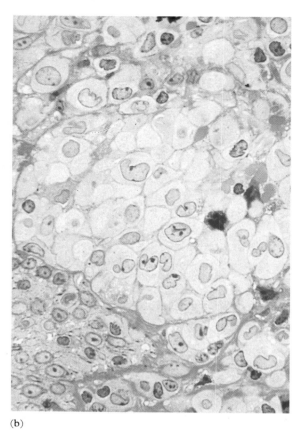

(b)

Fig. 22.12(a), (b) & (c). Letterer-Siwe Disease

This usually presents in infants as a papular rash (a), often with petechiae; the papules are brownish and may show scaling and crusting. The papules may be few in number, usually grouped, or can be very extensive; they are most common on face and scalp,

and when extensive they can involve much of the trunk. Unlike inflammatory skin disease, the lesions are fixed and do not go away. Subsequent systemic involvement is almost invariable.

Histologically, the infantile form shows a monotonous infiltrate of large histiocyte-like cells, usually in the

upper dermis and closely applied beneath the epidermal basement membrane. In scaling or crusting papules there is usually epidermal invasion. The cells have abundant pale eosinophilic cytoplasm and indented or reniform nuclei often with a linear groove. Micrograph (b) shows a very high magnification picture of typical cells expanding the papillary dermis and invading the epidermis, in a 1 μm resin section stained by Toluidine Blue. Electron microscopy in (c) shows that many of the cells contain occasional structures (arrows) resembling ill-formed Birbeck granules (inset), as seen in Langerhans cells (see Fig. 3.8). In older children and young adults, these cells form only a proportion of the infiltrate, the remainder being lymphocytes, eosinophils, histiocytic giant cells and occasional plasma cells; this probably represents a transitional form to Hand-Schüller-Christian disease and the prognosis is less grave.

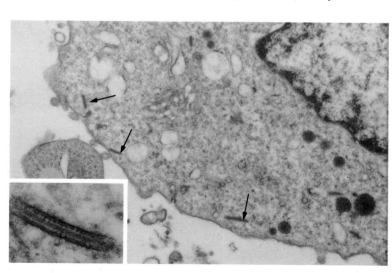

Table 22.1   Immunocytochemical markers in lymphoma

CD. No.	Specificity	Common antibodies
CD1	Cortical thymocytes, Langerhans cells	Nal/34, OKT 6
CD2	Sheep erythrocyte receptor, Pan-peripheral T cell marker	OKT 11, Leu 5
CD3	T cell receptor, Pan-peripheral T cell marker	OKT 3, UCHT 1
CD4	Helper T cell subset marker (Class II antigen assoc T cells)	OKT 4, Leu 3a
CD5	Pan T cell (some B cells, especially BCLL)	DKT 1, Leu 1
CD7	Pan T cell (Absent in CTCL)	3A 1, Dako T2
CD8	Suppressor T cell marker (Class 1 antigen assoc T cells)	OKT 8, Leu 2A
CD19/20/21	General B-cell markers	
CD22	Pan B cell	TO15, Dako pan-B
CD25	Interleukin 2 receptor	Anti Tac, Tu 69, Dako IL 2/R
CD45R	Pan B and T cell markers	MB1, MT1
—	Surface immunoglobulin	K & L light chain GMDA & E heavy chain
—	Dendritic reticulum cell markers	E 11, ORC 1

CD No.: Cluster of differentiation number.
From Reinherz EL et al 1986 International workshop on leucocyte typing II. Springer Verlag.

23.   Fibrous and fibrohistiocytic tumours and proliferations

Introduction

There are a number of lesions in the skin which were formerly thought to be derived entirely from fibroblasts, but it is now clear that these lesions contain cells having some of the structural and functional properties of histiocytes. Ultrastructural studies have also demonstrated a cell described as a myofibroblast within many of the tumour-like fibromatous proliferations; these spindle-shaped cells show cytoplasmic smooth muscle myofilaments as well as the abundant rough endoplasmic reticulum characteristic of fibroblasts. It is likely that many fibrohistiocytic new growths originate from a primitive mesenchymal cell, capable of differentiating into either a collagen-producing fibroblast or a phagocytic tissue histiocyte (or intermediate forms).

Illustrated and discussed in this chapter are a number of the fibrous and fibrohistiocytic tumours and proliferations which may present in the skin; many other conditions are manifest as subcutaneous masses or related to underlying joints and therefore present to general or orthopaedic surgeons.

The most commonly encountered lesions are those belonging to the *histiocytoma-dermatofibroma* group (see Fig. 23.1); these are now regarded as representing different ends of the spectrum of the same basic lesion. *Dermatofibrosarcoma protruberans* (Fig. 23.2) is a slow growing dermal tumour which behaves in a malignant fashion with local invasion, but progression is very slow and the tumour rarely metastasizes. *Malignant fibrous histiocytoma* (Fig. 23.3) is a sarcoma which most commonly occurs in the deep tissues of the thigh and buttock, but some appear to arise in subcutaneous tissue and may present as a skin tumour. The histogenetic relationship between dermatofibroma, dermatofibrosarcoma protruberans and malignant fibrous histiocytoma is not clear.

The term 'fibromatoses' is applied to a number of conditions characterized by irregular proliferation of fibrous tissue beneath the skin, probably originating in fascia. They are usually ill-defined and show a tendency to insinuate into normal adjacent tissue and hence may be difficult to excise adequately and permanently. Despite this apparent local invasive capacity, they are benign lesions and some spontaneously involute; such conditions include nodular pseudosarcomatous fasciitis and Dupuytren's contracture. Since they arise beneath the skin, these disorders are beyond the scope of this book.

There are some uncommon conditions which should be included in this chapter since recent electron microscopical and immunocytochemical studies have indicated that the predominant cell type involved in the proliferation is a histiocyte or histiocyte-related cell. Such tumour-like accumulations and proliferations include juvenile xanthogranuloma, reticulohistiocytic granuloma, multicentric reticulohistiocytosis and atypical fibroxanthoma.

Fig. 23.1(a)–(f). Histiocytoma-dermatofibroma
(illustrations opposite)

These lesions appear in the skin as hard brown-grey or flesh-coloured nodules that are round, smooth, 0.5–2.0 cm in diameter and slow-growing, and are commonest on the limbs in adults (a). Characteristically they submerge below the surface when squeezed, producing a dimple, though this physical sign is not specific.

Histologically, the lesions usually have two cell types: (i) small, compactly arranged fibroblasts with spindle-shaped nuclei and scanty cytoplasm, and (ii) histiocytes which usually have prominent pale-staining cytoplasm full of lipid (arrow in (c)). Sometimes the latter cells predominate to produce a mass with a yellowish cut face because of the large quantity of lipid; this variant is sometimes called histiocytoma cutis (d). Much more often the fibroblastic component predominates and the histiocytic cells are present as small scattered clumps. The spindle-shaped fibroblasts are tightly packed and arranged in complex whorled patterns (e), with variable amounts of intervening collagen which follows the lines laid down by the cells. Sometimes the amount of collagen is greatly increased and the cellularity of the lesions appears proportionately reduced (f). This loss of cellularity may highlight the large numbers of blood vessels present, some of which may be thick-walled; this variant is sometimes known inaccurately as sclerosing haemangioma and usually contains moderate amounts of haemosiderin. It is characteristic of this group of lesions that the edges of the lesion are indistinct laterally and deeply, with cells insinuating themselves between the collagen bundles of the normal dermis and down into subcutaneous fat. Despite this apparent local infiltration, the lesions are benign. The upper border is also ill-defined but is almost always separated from the overlying epidermis by some normal loose papillary dermis. The overlying epidermis is almost always thickened, with acanthosis, elongation of rete ridges and hyperkeratosis; there is often increased melanin pigmentation in the basal layer of the epidermis. Rarely, there may be focal basal cell hyperplasia mimicking early basal cell carcinoma.

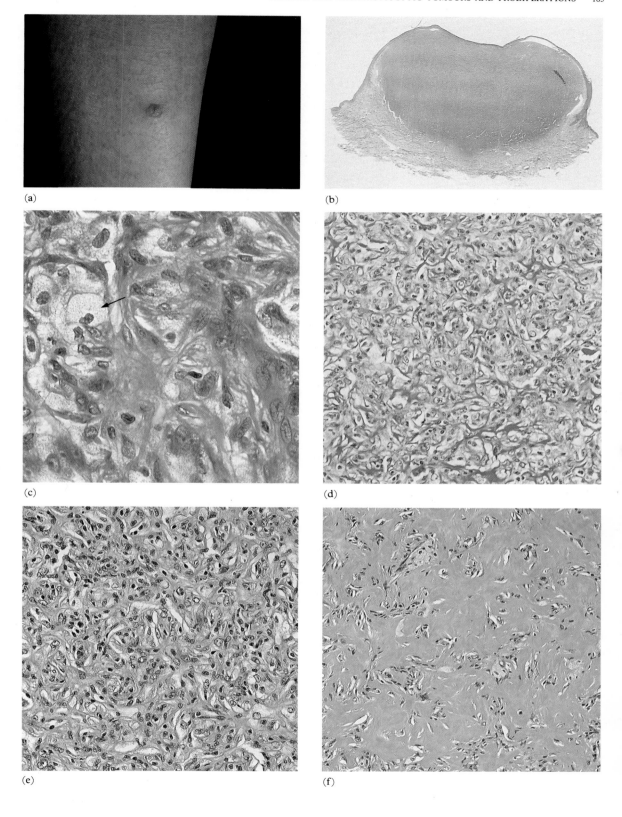

(a)

(b)

(c)

(d)

(e)

(f)

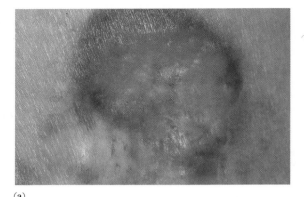

(a)

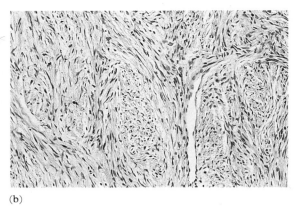

(b)

Fig. 23.2(a) & (b). Dermatofibrosarcoma protruberans

This slow-growing tumour usually presents on the trunk in adults as a smooth, firm, painless nodule which looks initially like a dermatofibroma but which slowly increases in size. Over several years it results in a hard, domed, flesh-coloured or pink telangiectatic plaque (a); this can evolve into a more protruberant lesion which may eventually ulcerate.

Histologically, the tumour is composed of spindle cells arranged in a fasciculated and whorled pattern, with various amounts of intervening collagen (b). At the periphery of the lesion, and particularly near the surface, the tumour can be histologically indistinguishable from dermatofibroma. However, at its centre the tumour is considerably more cellular and is composed of tightly packed fibroblast-like cells arranged in a storiform pattern, with little intervening collagen; similar cellular tumour is seen at the deepest margin where it infiltrates subcutaneous fat. It is vital that a substantial incision biopsy be taken, to include this characteristically cellular central area, otherwise an erroneous diagnosis of dermatofibroma may be made.

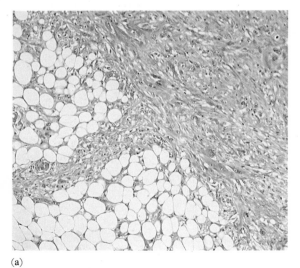

(a)

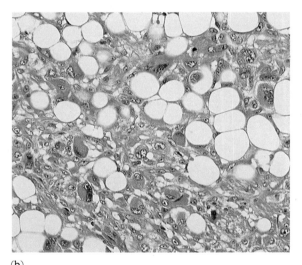

(b)

Fig. 23.3(a) & (b). Malignant fibrous histiocytoma

Lesions tend to present in skin as smooth, firm, reddish nodules which usually enlarge slowly. When growth is rapid, they ulcerate and bleed, and spread extensively both locally and via the blood stream.

Histologically, malignant fibrous histiocytoma shows spindle cells arranged in a fasciculated and whorled pattern, but in a variable and disorganized manner (a). The cells show considerable nuclear and cytoplasmic pleomorphism, and mitoses are frequent and often bizarre. Large multinucleate giant cells are frequent in some areas (b). Foci of haemorrhage and myxoid degeneration are common, as are scattered inflammatory cells, often mast cells. Although most of the tumour cells are spindle-shaped and fibroblast-like, a few histiocytes are seen, and electron microscopy shows a number of cell forms intermediate between fibroblasts and histiocytes.

Epithelioid sarcoma is rare, but is important because it can mimic granuloma annulare clinically and, less frequently, histologically. It presents as dermal or subcutaneous nodules, often grouped. The varying levels of the lesions in the skin, their disposition and colour, may help to distinguish them from granuloma annulare. Because they often arise near tendon sheath they may spread linearly; usual sites are forearm and lower leg.

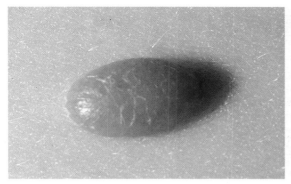

(a)

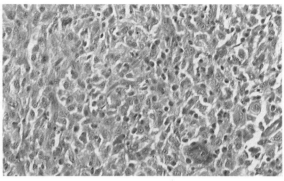

(b)

Fig. 23.4(a) & (b). Juvenile xanthogranuloma

These lesions (formerly called naevoxanthoendothelioma) usually occur as raised yellowish or red nodules (a) in the skin of infants or older children; they are occasionally present at birth. They may be single or multiple, and are usually less than 1 cm in diameter, although occasionally very large lesions, which tend to have a depressed centre, can occur. They usually gradually diminish in size within the first year of life and ultimately disappear.

Histologically, they are composed of large lipid-filled histiocytes with a variable infiltration of other cells including lymphocytes, eosinophils, histiocytes lacking lipid, and multinucleate Touton giant cells with a ring of nuclei arranged at the periphery of the cell. Small or early nodules may be almost entirely composed of lipid-filled histiocytes with little in the way of other cells, whereas older lesions usually show an abundant infiltration of other cells. Involuting lesions become less cellular and more fibroblastic with increasing collagen deposition.

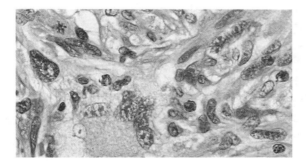

Fig. 23.5. Atypical fibroxanthoma

This is now regarded as a low-grade malignant fibrohistiocytic neoplasm of the skin, but with a good prognosis because of its superficial location, slow growth and tendency to metastasize late. It occurs most frequently as small raised nodule, usually less than 2 cm diameter on the face or neck of elderly men, but can occur in other sites, particularly in young people. Small lesions are covered by normal skin, but larger lesions show central ulceration.

The lesion shows histological similarities with malignant fibrous histiocytoma, being composed of variably pleomorphic cells, both polygonal and spindle cells, with scattered, swollen, foamy cells containing lipid droplets (hence the term fibroxanthoma); sometimes the lipid-filled cells are multinucleate giant cells, closely resembling Touton giant cells. An invariable finding is the presence of numerous multinucleate giant cells, many of which show marked nuclear pleomorphism. Although largely dermal, the tumour extends to the lower border of the epidermis and downwards into subcutaneous fat. At its deep and lateral borders the tumour is ill-defined, with fingers of tumour cells insinuating themselves into subcutaneous fat and normal dermal collagen.

Two rarely seen but histologically interesting histiocytic lesions in the skin are *reticulohistiocytic granuloma* and *multicentric reticulohistiocytosis*. These lesions are histologically virtually identical but clinically distinct. Reticulohistiocytic granuloma presents as smooth pale nodules, rarely larger tham 1 cm diameter, on the head and neck in adults. The lesion is usually solitary, but occasionally two or three may occur. Multicentric reticulohistiocytosis presents with large numbers of nodules scattered around the skin but tending to be most numerous on face, neck and hands. The nodules may be up to 2–3 cm in diameter but most are smaller; when very numerous and concentrated they may fuse together. There is almost always an associated arthritis, and the synovium of affected joints shows accumulation of cells similar to those seen in the skin. In both cases, spontaneous involution of the skin nodules is the rule, but this may be slow, particularly in multicentric reticulohistiocytosis.

Histologically, the lesions are composed of large histiocytes with pale eosinophilic cytoplasm, many of which are multinucleate. The large multinucleate giant cells are unlike those Touton giant cells seen in juvenile xanthogranuloma: the nuclei are irregularly arranged throughout the cytoplasm rather than arranged peripherally. There is an associated infiltrate of lymphocytes with some neutrophils, eosinophils and mast cells. Progressive fibrosis occurs in involuting lesions.

24. Miscellaneous tumours in the skin

Smooth muscle tumours

Leiomyomas in the skin may be derived from arrector pili muscle, when they usually appear as multiple red, raised dermal nodules 0.5–1.5 cm across, and are often tender, and sometimes painful; they are commonest on the trunk and limbs. Dartoic myoma is a solitary leiomyoma of the scrotum, labia or nipple, arising from the smooth muscle beneath the skin in these areas. Angioleiomyoma is a flesh-coloured dermal nodule 1–2 cm in diameter, usually on the lower leg, arising from the smooth muscle cells in the walls of blood vessels, usually veins. In the latter, some evidence of the vessel from which they have arisen can usually be seen in the tumour nodule, particularly if a connective tissue stain (e.g. elastic-van Gieson) is used.

Tumours derived from adipocytes

Lipomas are common in the subcutaneous fatty tissue and are usually 1–5 cm in diameter, soft, mobile, rubbery and lobulated. When multiple they may be associated with other lesions, e.g. neurofibromatosis and Gardner's syndrome. Adipose tissue is a major component of most mixed connective tissue hamartomas and congenital malformations in the skin, usually in subcutis. It may be found in association with haphazardly organized vascular channels (angiolipoma), with an admixture of fibrous and occasionally smooth muscle tissue. Angiolipomas are clinically like lipomas, but are painful.

Tumours of nerve sheath origin

Neurofibroma is a complex benign tumour or hamartoma composed of mainly Schwann cells, but with elements of endoneurium and perineurium and axons present. They may occur singly, or in large numbers as part of von Recklinghausen's neurofibromatosis.

    Neurilemmoma (schwannoma) is a benign tumour of the Schwann cells of a peripheral nerve and is located in the subcutis.

    Neuromas are complex tumour-like masses of nerves arranged haphazardly, with thick perineurial sheaths, embedded in collagen. Most are post-traumatic in origin and solitary, but they may be multiple and associated with one of the groups of multiple endocrine neoplasia.

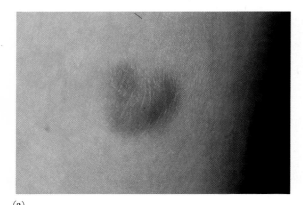

(a)

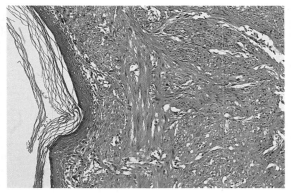

(b)

Fig. 24.1(a) & (b). Leiomyoma
The clinical photograph shows the typical naked-eye appearance of a skin leiomyoma; the lesion is a raised red nodule approximately 1 cm across (a). The red colour suggests a dermal location and an origin from arrector pili. They are composed of compact interlacing bundles of smooth muscle cells (b), and may be located in either the dermis or the subcutis. Dermal lesions are probably derived from either the smooth muscle of arrector pili muscles

(piloleiomyomas) or from the wall of dermal veins (angioleiomyomas), whilst those in the subcutaneous tissue are all derived from veins. In leiomyoma originating from vessel wall, the tumour mass contains a number of vessels, which can be easily seen on a connective tissue stain such as a Van Gieson; often the large vein from which the tumour has arisen can be identified. The connective tissue stain also reveals that the smooth muscle is embedded in collagenous fibrous tissue.

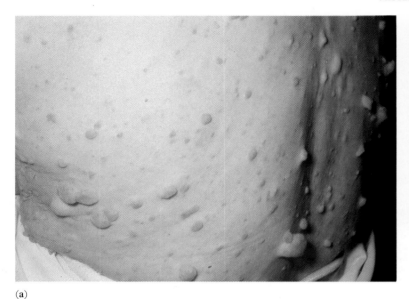

(a)

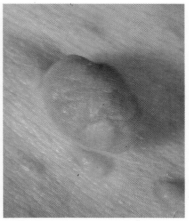

(b)

**Fig. 24.2(a), (b) & (c).
Neurofibroma**

Clinically, neurofibromas in the skin appear as soft, fleshy, raised lesions which are often pedunculated (b). In the inherited disorder of von Recklinghausen's disease, they are present in very large numbers both in the skin (a) and internal organs. They occasionally appear as rubbery plaques (plexiform neurofibroma). A striking feature is that they can be invaginated into the skin by finger pressure. They are mainly located in the dermis and are usually well-defined although not encapsulated; larger tumours extend into the upper subcutis. They are composed of spindle-shaped cells embedded in wavy reticulin and collagen fibres (c). Mast cells are common, and mucinous or myxomatous secondary change is so frequent that some degree is almost invariable. Abnormal nerve fibres (arrow) may be seen within the tumour, and sometimes entering it at one side; they are best demonstrated with special nerve or connective tissue stains.

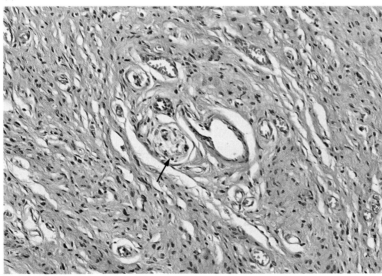

(c)

Fig. 24.3. Neurilemmoma

These uncommon solitary tumours are usually subcutaneous rather than in the skin. They occur close to the peripheral nerve from which they develop. They are usually pink or flesh-coloured nodules which may be intradermal or subcutaneous, and are often painful. Histologically, they are usually well-circumscribed with a variable fibrous capsule; the tumour is composed of elongated spindle cells (Schwann cells) which are either tightly packed (Antoni type A pattern) or loosely separated and oedematous (Antoni type B pattern). A common feature is the arrangement of the spindle-shaped nuclei into regular compact rows (palisading). Rows of palisaded nuclei are sometimes parallel to each other, with loose acellular material between two rows. This change occurs within the Antoni A pattern; cystic changes may occur within Antoni B tissue. In contrast to neurofibroma, nerve fibres are rarely seen in neurilemmoma.

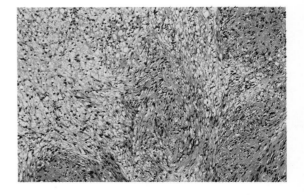

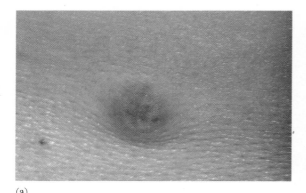

(a)

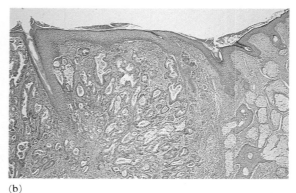

(b)

Fig. 24.4(a) & (b). Metastatic carcinoma

Blood-borne or lymphatic metastasis of an internal carcinoma to the skin is quite uncommon, although local recurrence of mammary carcinoma in the skin of the anterior chest following partial or total mastectomy is more common. In men, the most common carcinoma to spread to skin is carcinoma of the bronchus, usually oat-cell type; in women, breast is the most common, even excluding those involving skin by direct invasion or local recurrence.

The clinical appearance of metastatic carcinoma depends on whether the tumour is present within blood vessels, lymphatics or as diffuse or discrete nodular infiltration of the dermis. Other factors affecting the appearance depend on factors such as the nature of the tumour, the quantity present, and the degree of fibrous stromal reaction to the presence of tumour cells. The latter is particularly marked in metastatic mammary carcinoma (carcinoma-en-cuirasse).

In the photomicrograph, islands of metastatic colonic adenocarcinoma are present in upper dermis in vulva.

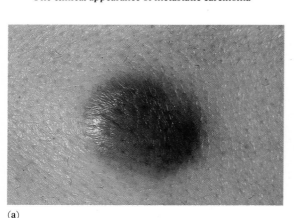

(a)

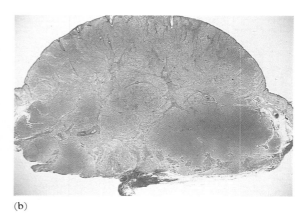

(b)

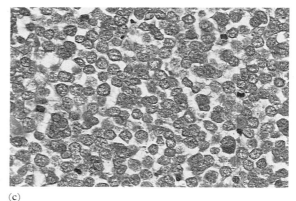

(c)

Fig. 24.5(a), (b) & (c). Merkel cell tumour

This unusual tumour is believed to originate from the Merkel cells in the epidermis (see p. 18). They most commonly present as a solitary red nodule (a), usually on the face or neck of elderly people. Both at low magnification (b) and at higher magnification (c), the tumorous infiltration of the epidermis closely resembles that seen in some types of B cell lymphoma. The tumour cells are small and round or polygonal, and darkly staining as a result of a high nucleus/cytoplasm ratio. They are tightly packed with little or no intervening stroma; at the edges the tumour cells may grow out in cords. Cytological distinction from malignant lymphoid cells may depend on immunocytochemistry or electron microscopy. Ultrastructurally, the scanty cytoplasm of the Merkel cells contain small numbers of membrane-bound secretory granules indicative of the neuroendocrine nature of the Merkel cell, and the cells show immunocytochemical reactivity for S100, NSE, PGP9.5, but are negative for LCA (leucocyte common antigen), which is almost invariably positive in lymphoma.

Index